Honour Due

The Story of Dr. Leonora Howard King

Margaret Negodaeff-Tomsik

Association médicale canadienne
Canadian Medical Association

Edited by Edwinna von Baeyer

Consultants:
Jacalyn Duffin, MD, PhD, FRCPC, Kingston, Ontario
James A. Leith, FRSC, Kingston, Ontario
Rev. S. Derek Shelly, BA, MDiv, Almonte, Ontario

Canadian Cataloguing in Publication Data

Negodaeff-Tomsik, Margaret, 1950–
Honour due : the story of Dr. Leonora Howard King

Includes bibliographical references and index.
ISBN 0-920169-33-3

1. King, Leonora Howard, 1851–1925. 2. Women physicians–China–biography. 3. Missionaries, Medical–China–Biography. 4. Women physicians–Canada–Biography. 5. Missionaries, Medical–Canada–Biography. I. Title.

R722.32.K55N44 1999 610.69'5'092 C99-900157-4

Published by
Canadian Medical Association
1867 Alta Vista Drive
Ottawa ON K1G 3Y6
Canada

Printed in Canada

Association médicale canadienne
Canadian Medical Association

Honour thy physician with the honour due
… for the uses which ye may have … .

— *Ecclesiasticus 38:1*

Foreword

The story of Dr. Leonora Howard King goes far beyond that of a woman's struggle to enter a profession denied to her solely on the basis of her sex. It is also the story of an incredible life, a story that was almost lost by the passage of time.

When the author first brought this story to our attention, our first reaction was disbelief. How could the story of the first Canadian doctor to work in China, a woman who was made a Mandarin by the Empress Dowager of China, be unknown to the Canadian Medical Association? How could a life described by a contemporary as "something out of *The Arabian Nights*" be totally unknown to the Canadian public? And yet it was true.

Denial of entrance to medical school in Canada meant much more to this young woman than simply going to the United States to get a degree. It meant that her remarkable achievements were overlooked by the Canadian medical community.

It is with great pleasure that the Canadian Medical Association now publishes *Honour Due: The Story of Dr. Leonora Howard King*. This ensures that Leonora Howard King's life story finally becomes part of our Canadian history and heritage.

Susan Swiggum, MD, BSc, FRCP, Chair
Women Physicians' Issues Committee, CMA

Ian Warrack, MB, ChB, CCFP, Chair
Board of Directors, CMA

Preface

Dear Reader:

I am not a professional biographer. I am not religious. I am not a physician. And I am not an academic. Were I any of the above, one might begin to get a dim idea of why I have now spent six years researching an obscure missionary doctor who practised in China in the 19th century. Suffice it to say, I do not always have my marbles.

Some of the blame must be laid upon my husband, Stephen Nicholas George Tomsik, who has a passion for rescuing old books from obscurity or worse. Having been well trained to bring me a cuppa in bed of a Saturday morning, one day in 1993, he presented me both with a cup of tea and one of his rescued books. This book was a turn-of-the-century type of Canadian women's *Who's Who*. It contained 354 photo-plates and one-paragraph biographies of everyone from the Countess of Durham, wife of the High Commissioner and Governor General of British North America in 1838, to Mrs. Laura Secord, who saved this country from American attack.

While sipping tea and flipping pages, I came across one name that made me stop, simply because female physicians were few and far between way back then. After reading the biographical paragraph, I yelled to poor Stephen, who was quietly enjoying his morning paper. "Somebody has to DO something for this woman!" I cried, tea spilling on the sheets. "No one's ever heard of her. She was a true hero!" We looked at each other. "Oops," I said.

Thus began what was at times very tedious, at times enormously exciting, research into the life of Dr. Leonora Howard King. Luck has been with me in uncanny quantities throughout these six years, prompting many to say "this book wants to be written, and Leonora wants you to write it."

The first stroke of luck was that Leonora was born within driving distance of Ottawa, where I live. The second was that Ottawa houses the National

Archives, which provided me with birth and death records of Leonora's family and St. Joseph's University, which has an excellent set of missionary records. The third and most important piece of fortune was finding out that Ron Howard, Leonora's great-nephew, still lives in Athens, Ontario, formerly Farmersville, where my subject was born. From Ron to his sister Gwen Conerly, to her cousins Geraldine and Dorothy, I began to get a small but beautiful picture of Leonora's life.

But one cannot do this kind of research without dollars. I managed to obtain a grant from the marvellous Canada Council, and armed with the lolly I made it all the way to China, and then to less-exotic but definite treasure troves at the Day Missions Library, Yale University, and Victoria University in Toronto.

What you are about to read is not fiction. At times I wish I had decided upon a "historical novel," which would have been far easier! In any case, I hope the scenes and the people will come as much to life for you as they did for me.

Sincerely
Margaret Negodaeff-Tomsik

Acknowledgements

Where does one begin? With my treasured husband, Stephen Tomsik, who found an old book with a picture of Leonora and one lonely paragraph about her life? With friends at the National Press Club, who coached me on how to write a proposal for a grant? How about the very helpful woman at the Chinese Embassy who helped me plan my trip! Of course, one cannot even begin to thank the person responsible for publication, Dr. Cathy Younger-Lewis, publishing consultant to the Canadian Medical Association. Like a Shih Tzu with a bone, Dr. Younger-Lewis wouldn't let me quit. As I write this, she is probably pacing up and down, wondering if I'm ever going to finish.

I am very grateful to the Canada Council, without whose generous grant I could not have researched this book. I would also specifically like to thank my long-suffering bank manager, Tom Gaul, for believing in me. Then there is the Department of Foreign Affairs, who put me through to Tang Yannan at our Embassy in China, who in turn put me in touch with Wang Yi at the International Culture Exchange Agency of Tianjin. Yu Yong, also known as Barbara Yu, was my guide in Tianjin, and she was nothing short of wonderful. Writers and historians Liu Jiantang and Du Wenping of Tianjin were of great help by sending me more information and books on the Astor Hotel and the churches of Tianjin.

Many thanks to Martha Lund Smalley, curator of the Day Missions Library at Yale University, and to Susan M. Eltscher, assistant general secretary, General Commission on Archives and History, United Methodist Church, in Madison, New Jersey. Also of assistance were Lauralee A. Ensign of the University of Michigan's Alumni Records office, Ruth Dyck Wilson, reference coordinator at the United Church Archives, Victoria University, University of

Toronto, and Mrs. R.E. Seton, archivist at the School of Oriental and African Studies at the University of London, UK. My appreciation also to the librarians at Ottawa's St. Joseph University.

Leonora Howard King's family were of tremendous assistance. While searching birth records at the National Archives, I found great-nephew Ron Howard still living in Athens, Ontario, Leonora's original home. Ron put me onto his sister, Gwen Conerly, who lives in Florida. A tremendously enthusiastic Gwen got in touch with her cousins, Geraldine and Dorothy (Tay) Howard, in Toronto, who showed me prized memorabilia, reminisced about their great-aunt Leonora, who they had met when they were children, and put together a wonderful set of photographs. Mrs. Grace Howard also kindly furnished valuable photographs for this book. Mrs. Lois Schroeder of Frankville, Ontario, helped me with preliminary research in Athens, formerly Farmersville, where Leonora was born.

My father-in-law, John von Hunnius, enabled me to understand a bit of Beijing by arranging for me to meet Xing Lijun, now Julie Xing, who became a good friend on both sides of the Pacific. In Ottawa, dear Denny and Elizabeth Tang helped me with translation and with travelling in China. Press Club member Gord Cullingham introduced me to Beijing doctor Yuning Wu, who had done her residency at the Ottawa Civic Hospital, and who introduced me to the "real" China, including those wonderful noodles at the night market. Paul Delahanty, who for a time acted as my agent, was a tremendous help and must be acknowledged as original editor of my Introduction. Tom Sloan lent me his Chinese-English dictionaries and tapes, which I have yet to return! Jim Moore and Charles Morrow listened to me and discussed my book for years. Dear friend Susan Barnabé put up with my thoughts, doubts and occasional moments of insanity with considerable aplomb and loyalty. Don Gollan, James Pope and Osman Siddiqui held my hands and bought me wine. Marilyn Ronald's home in Hamilton, Ontario, has remained my oasis, lo these many writing years. Margaret Stone and Brian Linklater gave me their unbiased comments, for which I am eternally grateful.

Last but certainly not least, bouquets to my stalwart and excellent editor, Edwinna von Baeyer, who, through nasty bouts of bronchitis, stroked my shivering little ego while pointing out repetitions, lousy punctuation, and the fact that I sometimes spelled a word three different ways.

This book is dedicated not only to Leonora herself but to all the forgotten women of the last century, including the Lady (Vicereine) Li, wife of Li Hung-chang, who not only was responsible for Leonora's medical success but was also an intelligent philanthropist who remained a close personal friend and protector for many turbulent years. It is dedicated to Leonora's husband, Alex King, who stayed resolutely by her side in China when he would have preferred to retire (probably on a lecture tour!), in Canada or in England. It is dedicated to young girls the world over who wonder about careers in the sciences, the adventure of travel, and the challenge of the unknown.

A warm message of "youyi" (friendship) and tremendous thanks (xie xie!) goes out to my hosts in China, some of whom also became my good friends. I hope my small amount of research on your great country is somewhat accurate — if not, please forgive this "long-nosed Westerner!"

Bless you all.

Introduction

In the 19th century, thousands of westerners travelled to China to spread the Christian gospel. Many were motivated by simple goodness, while others saw fantastic opportunities for adventure, and ultimately gained great power and wealth. A few were successful in their original intents and their legacies still flourish. Many others were killed or tortured for their efforts, died of fever, or were ordered home for their own safety.

Almost without fail, the China missionaries who returned wrote about their experiences or told their tales in cross-country lecture tours. Some told the truth as they saw it, which was not very popular with the home organizations. The behaviour of some Canadian missionaries after the Boxer Rising of 1900, for instance, resulted in banishment to remote outposts, away from hungry domestic newspaper reporters. Although this did not prevent the missionaries from writing their memoirs, publication was usually delayed until the whole outrage had become a distant memory. A number of the missionaries may, over the years, be forgiven obvious embellishment of their hazy moments of glory. Others have been proven outright liars. In any case, they are all dead now.

Few contemporary books have been written about the missionaries of the last century, and fewer still about the tens of thousands who happened to be women. This book is the story of one woman whose skill as a physician was surpassed only by her will to survive, and more remarkably, to remain stubbornly behind when hundreds of others fled. Her name was Leonora Howard King, the first Canadian to practise medicine in China.

Leonora was born in 1851, in Farmersville (now Athens), Ontario — a prosperous and pious farming community. She, like many other spinster farmgirls, became a teacher, responsible for the Leeds County district collection of one-room schoolhouses. However, medicine had a strong tradition in the Howard family. Although Leonora's father was a farmer, his father and two of his brothers were physicians. Living only a day's trip from Queen's University's School of Medicine at Kingston, Ontario,* it would have seemed an easy step for Leonora to follow her relatives' lead. But women were not allowed to study at Queen's medical school or, in fact, any Canadian medical school. Young Leonora had to venture south to the University of Michigan at Ann Arbor, where she received her MD, in 1876.

Even then, Leonora was unable to practise medicine in Canada. Doctors with MDs from the United States were required to do a course at a Canadian medical school. Leonora, as a woman, was not allowed to attend any medical classes in Canada.

It should be noted that a member of Leonora's local church had held the distinction of being the first Canadian woman to live in China (with her American missionary husband). It is probable that Leonora had heard Mrs. Virgil Hart speak on the need for missionaries in China, or that she had read the Harts' reports of life in that far-off land. Whether it was Mrs. Hart's example of self-sacrifice or, and this is more likely, the idea of exotic adventure that attracted Leonora, we will also never know. The decision meant going to the other side of the world, leaving behind family and friends, knowing she might never see them again. But this decision started her on, in the words of one 19th-century lady, "a life that reads like a story from *The Arabian Nights*."

Finding that she was unable to practise professionally with even the fledgling Canadian missionary groups, Leonora joined the American Methodist Episcopal Missionary Society, one emerging branch of which was the Woman's Foreign Missionary Society (WFMS). She was sent to China in 1877, at age 26.

The news of Leonora's skill as a physician quickly spread throughout North China, for reasons you are about to discover. By 1884, the young doctor had single-handedly created a practice devoted entirely to Chinese women and children — a remarkable feat in a country where women were held in contempt. The missionary societies at home were overjoyed at this triumph. They were not as delighted when Leonora left the WFMS upon her marriage to Rev. Alexander King (London Missionary Society). Although she still worked with physicians from her husband's and other missionary societies, Leonora Howard King was, from that time on, supported almost exclusively by the Chinese.

Friend of royalty and the poor alike, Leonora taught Western medicine to and treated Chinese women and children for 47 years. She operated her hos-

*Kingston is now about one hour away from Athens. In those days, it would have taken about a day by horse and buggy.

pitals from temples, back doors, broken-down inns, and finally good "modern" facilities. She stubbornly continued through flood, famine, many anti-foreign movements and two major wars. As the first female recipient of the Ch'ing court's Order of the Double Dragon, she was for a short time well-known both in China and at home. Then, like other women of the times, she was forgotten.

A Final Note of Explanation

For consistency with the times, the City of Beijing will from now on be called by its old name of Peking, and Leonora's home, now known as Tianjin, will be Tientsin. Chihli province, containing the treaty port of Tientsin, no longer exists, but is referred to frequently in the text. The modern seaside resort of Beidahe is referred to by its old name of Peitaiho. China, to the Chinese, is also known as the Middle Kingdom, and the various emperors were called Sons of Heaven. The great Li Hongzhang, the former Viceroy of Chihli Province, is known by his old name of Li Hung-chang. For an interpretation of other 19th-century names and their new incarnations, please refer to the list in the back of the book. Finally, it would be difficult to talk about foreigners in China without giving the reader some historical background. With your permission, then, we will embark upon a short historical tour of the four major efforts to evangelize China in the name of Christianity.

By 1877, when young Leonora Howard arrived in Peking, the Chinese had been dealing with evangelists for centuries. The oldest solid record refers to the trader Alopen, who appeared at the court of Emperor T'ai Tsung of in AD 635. A beautifully carved statue, unearthed in 1625 in a village near Sian (Xian), shows two mythical beasts holding a precious pearl, coupled with a cross surmounting a lotus and a cloud. The heading reads "A Monument to the Diffusion throughout the Middle Kingdom of the Illustrious Teaching of Ta Ch'in" (thought to be Syria). The tablet summarizes the Christian faith, albeit in distinctly Chinese terms.

Alopen oddly enough crops up again in 781. At this time the Son of Heaven [T'ai Tsung's son, the Emperor Kao Tsung], issued a proclamation commending the Christian doctrine to all. Kao Tsung, who seemed quite impressed with the theory, commanded that churches be built in all provinces and honour conferred on Alopen — or presumably, his memory. Kao Tsung also bestowed upon Alopen the title of "Bishop of the Great Law." Written in both Chinese and Syriac are the names of the clergy of the time, including the Patriarch of Seleuci-Ctesiphon in Mesopotamia, head of the Nestorian Church.

This initial success on the part of the Christian adventurers was short-lived.

By 845, Taoist monks had managed to have Christian, Buddhist and other religions brutally suppressed, if not wiped out.

Christianity re-emerged in the 13th century with the Franciscan John of Montecorvino, later to become an archbishop. John was the first Roman Catholic missionary in the Far East, arriving at the Mongol Court of Peking in 1295. His instructions from Pope Nicholas, to "bring back to the Christian faith the unbelieving peoples of the East and schismatic and erring Christians," were not very popular among some competitive Nestorians, who hindered his missionary activities fairly successfully. Although John was buried with great honours in 1328, his mission declined rapidly thereafter.

The Nestorians, on the other hand, forged ahead for a number of years. One Franciscan traveller noted that in the 1330s, more than 30,000 Nestorian Christians were living in China. Their existence was doomed when the conqueror Tamberlaine commenced a slaughter that lasted almost 50 years.

The final evangelistic effort began in 1552, when Francis Xavier, later canonized, turned to China after having spread his word in Goa, Japan, and many other places. He died that very first winter of a fever, unsuccessful in his efforts to gain entrance to Canton. But exactly 30 years later in Macao, the Jesuit scholar Matteo Ricci plunged into a serious study of the Mandarin language, a skill that helped him become the most famous missionary of his time. Ricci had a prodigious memory and an excellent command of mathematics — one area in which the literate, artistic Chinese were at the time sadly lacking. The monk produced for them a map of the world, diplomatically placing China, the "Middle Kingdom," in the centre.

Ricci also provided pictures of European architecture, clocks and other innovations as evidence that Westerners were not, as commonly thought by this ancient, cultured civilization, complete barbarians. In addition to learning Chinese at an astonishing rate, he, like many later missionaries, adopted Chinese dress and customs. When Ricci died in 1610, he had converted more than 300 people in Peking alone, and it is estimated that 2,000 more now resided elsewhere in the Middle Kingdom. It is probably safe to say that in 40 years, Ricci accomplished single-handedly what no latter-day missionary could hope to achieve in a century of preaching.

By 1644, after the powerful Manchus had replaced the crumbling Ming dynasty, the Catholics were temporarily thrown into prison. As fortune would have it, another mathematician, Father Verbiest, successfully challenged the accuracy of a calendar produced by the Chinese president of the Board of Astronomy. As a result, he was given the position himself and became quite friendly with the current Son of Heaven. Now the Jesuits really began to flourish, with 20 missionaries and 100,000 converts scattered over 11 provinces. But just to be on the safe side, the Emperor K'ang-hsi cautiously forbade the entry of new missionaries and the building of new churches. In 1692, he signed a Decree of the Board of Rites — predecessor of many similar agreements with the foreigners — that gave protection to Catholic churches and public preaching.

Ricci the Jesuit scholar had, in his lifetime, decided that Confucianism was a philosophy and not really a religion, and therefore it did not conflict with Christianity. This created a serious rift between the Dominicans and the Jesuits, who presented arguments to various Popes for an exhaustive period lasting from 1643 to 1706. The Chinese responded by saying that Ricci's most reasonable interpretation was the one that would stick, or else. The confrontation in Rome continued. In 1717, the inevitable happened: China missionaries were banished, their churches destroyed, and persecution broke out that lasted a century.[1]

Robert Morrison of the London Missionary Society was the first Protestant missionary in China, arriving at Canton in 1807. Morrison, who plunged into studying the language, made a tremendous contribution by translating most of the Bible into Chinese. But until 1842, the only part of the Middle Kingdom in which foreign merchants were permitted to set foot — and then only between October and March — was an area on the Canton waterfront. In that year Britain defeated China in what became known as the Opium War, in which the former claimed their right to import and traffick in that odious drug. Through the subsequent Treaty of Nanking, Europe gained entrance to significant areas of Chinese land. In 1844, the Wanghia Treaty was negotiated with the Americans, thus opening the door for many missionaries who had not had access to Chinese souls.[2] Under these and the later "unequal treaties," Western missionaries secured privileges all across China. These included extraterritorial rights, in which foreigners accused of offences, either against other foreigners or against Chinese themselves, would be tried in courts belonging to their own countries, rather than by Chinese law.

In the period covered by this book — 1870 to 1925 — China missions had become big business. The 1870s, the decade that saw young Leonora Howard become a medical missionary, witnessed in Christian countries, particularly among the middle classes, an odd fascination with evangelizing the world, or more simply, converting everyone to Christianity. Those who typically "received the call" were in the main small-town boys or, like Leonora, young spinsters brought up on the farm. Like Leonora, many had some higher education but not much urban sophistication. They most certainly had religious dedication, but there was also the delicious thought of spending their lives as champions of the Lord in mysterious, exotic surroundings.

Let us now, then, follow in the footsteps of a gentle, intelligent and dedicated woman who, through a combination of luck, skill and determination, would help change the lives of millions of her Chinese sisters and those of at least a few Westerners.

Endnotes

1. Hayward, Victor E.W. *Christians and China*. Belfast: Christian Journals Limited, 1974, pp. 5-15.
2. Fleming, Peter. *The Siege at Peking*. New York: Dorset Press, 1990, p. 25.

Chronology

1851	Leonora Annetta Howard, born April 17, near Farmersville, Ontario, Canada.
1871	Li Hung-chang appointed Viceroy of Chihli Province. Tientsin becomes the provincial capital.
1872	Accepted at University of Michigan Women's Medical College.
1873	Viceroy Tseng Kuo-fan dies in Nanking. Li Hung-chang erects a memorial temple in Tientsin.
1875	Leonora "adopted" by Woman's Foreign Missionary Society (WFMS). Dr. John Kenneth Mackenzie of the London Missionary Society arrives in China.
1876	Leonora graduates with honours from medical school.
1877	Sails to China from San Francisco. Arrives Peking.
1879	Summoned to attend Lady Li, Vicereine of Chihli Province. Lady Li is cured and Leonora given part of Tseng Kuo-fan's memorial temple. Opens first Chinese hospital for women and children. Mackenzie given the other half to treat men and boys.
1880	Alex King and his wife Elizabeth set sail for China.
1881	Leonora opens the Isabella Fisher Hospital for Women and Children. Mrs. Elizabeth King dies.
1884	Leonora marries Alex.
1885	Opens Government Hospital for Women and Children.
1886	First Canadian missionary, Reverend Jonathan Goforth, arrives in China.
1888	Reverend James Frazer Smith, MD, and a contingent of other Canadian missionaries set up in Honan Province.
1889	Empress Dowager Tz'u-hsi formally abdicates in favour of the Kuang-hsu Emperor.
1891	Leonora and Alex take a trip to Canada and to England. Anti-foreign riots occur close to Tientsin.
1894	Sino-Japanese war breaks out over Korea. Leonora treats Chinese casualties.
	Dr. Sun Yat-sen visits Li Hung-chang in Tientsin.

1895	Li Hung-chang signs Treaty of Shimonoseki. Leonora receives Order of the Double Dragon from the Empress Dowager.
1896	Li Hung-chang goes on a world tour that includes Canada.
1898	Emperor proclaims "Hundred Days of Reform Movement." Li Hung-chang dismissed from Tsungli Yamen. Empress Dowager imprisons Emperor and resumes control of China.
1899–1900	The Boxers rebel against foreign presence. Sieges of Tientsin and Peking.
1901	Viceroy Li Hung-chang dies.
1902	Alex on furlough in England and Scotland. Leonora in Vienna.
1904	Russians fight Japanese for possession of Manchuria. Empress Dowager Tz'u-hsi suffers a stroke.
1908	Leonora opens China's first Government Medical School for Women. General Yuan Shih-kai made supreme military and naval commander, then premier of China. Empress Dowager and Emperor die within a day of each other.
1911	Chinese revolution breaks out October 10.
	Sun Yat-sen elected provisional president of China.
1912	Inauguration of a new Chinese Republic, January 1.
	Child Emperor Pu Yi forced to abdicate.
	Sun Yat-sen resigns presidency. National assembly elects Yuan Shih-kai provisional president. Kuomintang inaugurated in August.
1913	Second revolution breaks out, led by Chiang Kai-shek and Chen Chih-mei. Kuomintang dissolved.
1915	Third revolution in Yunnan. WFMS opens a new Isabella Fisher Hospital. A room is named in honour of Leonora.
1916	Leonora and Alex officially retire.
	On January 1, Yuan Shih-kai becomes emperor. On March 22, he restores the republic. On June 6, he dies. Sun Yat-sen returns to China.
1917	China breaks off diplomatic relations with Germany, March 14. Bill promoting China's participation in world war presented to parliament, May 8. Pu Yi briefly restored to throne, July 1. China declares war on Germany and Austria, August 14. Sun Yat-sen elected generalissimo by parliament, September 1.
1919	May 4, students' movement. Sun Yat-sen resigns post. Various provincial wars.
1921	Sun Yat-sen elected president.
1922	War breaks out in Chihli province.
1923	Leonora and Alex visit relatives in Canada.
1924	Deposed Emperor Pu Yi forced to leave Forbidden City.
1925	Sun Yat-sen dies March 12, at age 60.
	Leonora Howard King dies June 30, at age 74.

Chapter one

Beginnings
1872

Go, and the Lord be with thee.
— I Samuel 17:37

The little town of Farmersville, now Athens, Ontario, rests in some of central Canada's finest farmland. In 1872, Peter Howard, gentleman farmer, kept a fine herd of dairy cows and an equally fine stable of horses. His gentle British-born wife, Dorothy Carter Howard, had borne him a son, Eugene Alamanzer, now 27, and Leonora Annetta, four years his junior. Eugene had blinded himself accidentally as a youth, but would go on, not only to take over his father's farm, but to serve several terms as a Member of Parliament. At age 23, Leonora, tall, grey eyed, reed slim and with a wonderful head of unruly red-gold hair, was a teacher responsible for schoolhouses stretching from County Leeds all the way to Vankleek Hill, more than 160 kilometres to the east.

Leonora's family had lived in this area for at least three generations. In 1802, Napolean Howard had purchased land at nearby Soperton for a cemetery plot. He then expanded his holdings, snapping up surrounding land at Glen Morris. Napolean's farm had passed into the hands of his nephew, Peter Gilton Howard, because he loved the land. Peter's uncles, cousins and siblings had headed for more urban climes to become doctors, lawyers and politicians.

The Howards were a large and sprawling family, as well-known for their civic activities as their ability to produce intelligent offspring. This branch had a long and aristocratic history dating back to the first dukes of Norfolk and Surrey. Leonora's grandfather, also named Peter, was a physician. He had married Sarah Munsall on Christmas Day, 1792. From 1794 to 1813, Peter and Sarah produced a total of eight boys, and one girl by the name of Mary Ann. Two of the boys died as children. Two others, William Wilkie and Alpheus Ruggles Howard, became physicians like their father. Peter Gilton Howard, Leonora's father, would continue the line of "the farming Howards."

The first Howard home at nearby Soperton was a lovely structure, two storeys high and twice as wide. Bricks for the house, from a brickworks in a field across the road, had been made of a thick blue clay, mixed with straw, that was then trampled by teams of oxen. The massive walls were built "three bricks thick," or about 38 centimetres in total. The sturdy timbers were hand-hewn, 30 to 36 centimetres across. In one corner of the property was a blockhouse that had been operated as a medical school by Leonora's uncle, Dr. Alpheus Howard, who would later move to the United States. The family loved to tell the story about Alpheus' role in the dissection of the first man hanged at the Brockville jail (Brockville is 35 kilometres from Soperton). Apparently Alpheus managed to talk a jailer into relinquishing the body of a man named Simpson, hanged for murder. The body was smuggled home hidden in a spring wagon. Alpheus' medical students dissected the body for their studies. The family preserved the skeleton for many years.

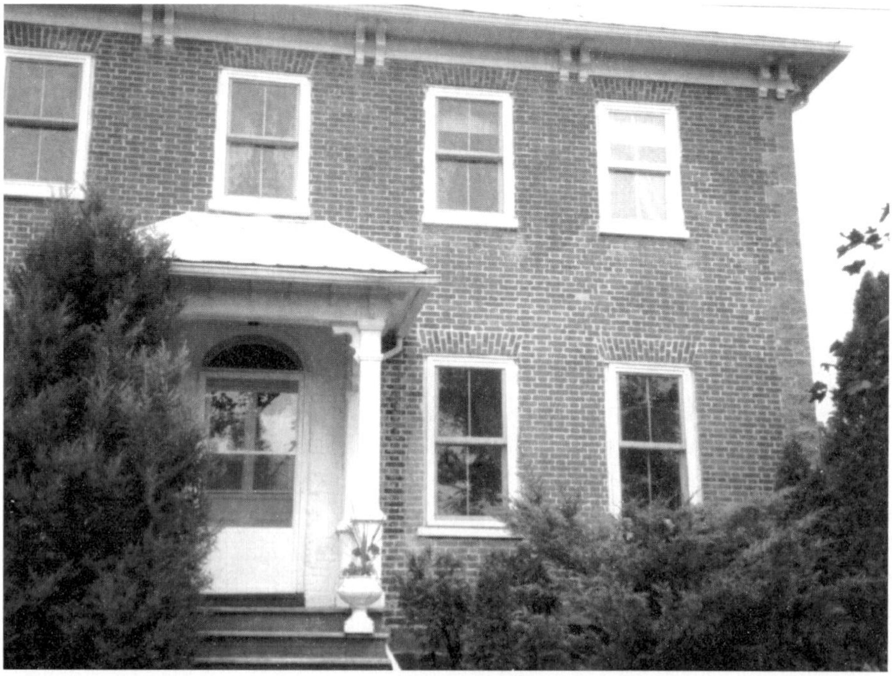

The Howard homestead, Soperton, Ontario

Although she had first settled on a career as a teacher, Leonora wanted desperately to be a doctor. Like other women before her, she had first tried to gain acceptance at the Royal College of Physicians and Surgeons in nearby Kingston, and like those others, she had failed miserably in her efforts. No lady, they had decided, would risk her delicate constitution, not to mention her reputation, by exposing herself to human body parts, and heaven forbid, male body parts. Even now, with qualified women returning with degrees earned in the United States, the professors and the young men they taught still refused to tolerate the thought of women entering their rarefied, almost godlike, atmosphere.

For women, life in the late 19th century was alternately exciting and tedious: exciting because many avenues of education were opening up, and tedious because Victorian conventions had to be observed. Leonora was brought up in a strict Methodist family. More women than men respected the Sabbath, probably because church was the main centre of social life. Men attended church, but also spent the Sabbath puttering around the house, fishing, hunting, and for some, playing cards, playing billiards, and drinking.

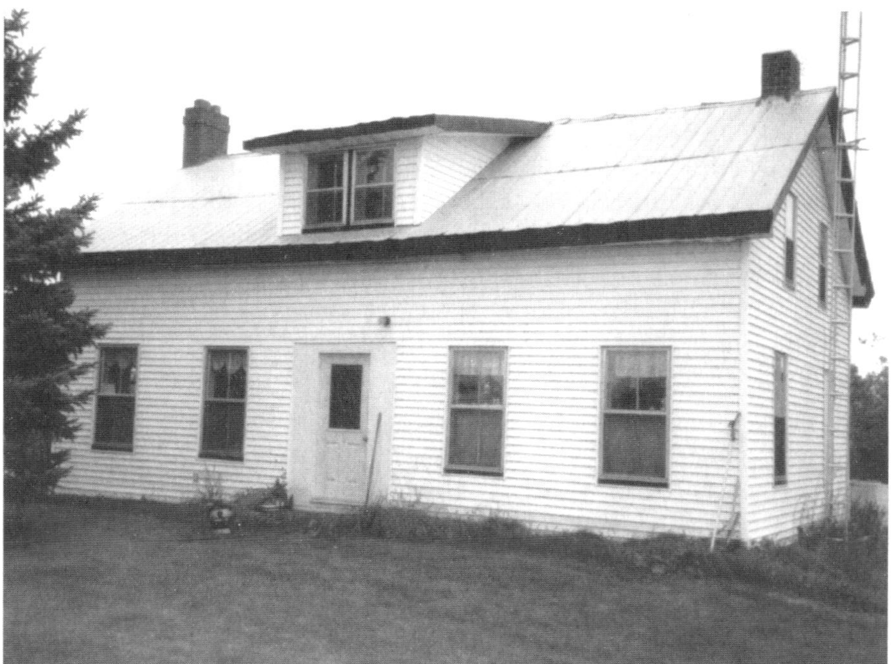

The farmhouse at Athens, Ontario

Living in a farming community, Leonora would have met young men by attending dances, particularly at weddings, barn raisings, and husking bees. Songfests were also popular, with traditional British folk songs such as *Barbara Allen*, and American imports like *Old Folks at Home*, or *Oh! Susannah*. In Upper Canada, later to be the Province of Ontario, fiddle and harmonica music was most popular, followed by the more genteel sounds of the pianoforte. In winter, everyone enjoyed sleigh rides. Those who were courting could snuggle under a buffalo robe and at least hold hands. Berrying, attending lectures, and walking home from church socials were also ways to "date."

Like any small community, the populace of Soperton and Farmersville liked to socialize with each other. Leonora's extended family would often gather to eat together, sing, play games, and talk about the latest books. Amateur theatre was popular. Shows were performed in churches, and tents in summertime. The works of Shakespeare were always playing somewhere, but *Uncle Tom's Cabin* was extremely popular with religious families.

Leonora Howard was not beautiful. Her height, her willowy figure and wonderful hair, her serious grey eyes and overly generous mouth did not quite add up to the Victorian ideal of fragile beauty. We know nothing of Leonora's early love life, but suffice it to say that during this time, women looked at marriage as bringing "some joys, but many crosses." One of those crosses was that women were not supposed to enjoy lovemaking, even within marriage. In 1870, a Dr. George Napheys wrote in his *Transmission of Life*: "The best mothers, wives, and managers of households know little or nothing of the sexual pleasure. Love of home, children and domestic duties are the only pleasures they feel."

Had Leonora married in her neighbourhood, she would have had an average of five to seven children, and been saddled with endless sewing, mending, cooking and cleaning. Any freedom brought by her income as a schoolteacher would have abruptly disappeared, because she would now depend on her husband for support. Only spinsters were allowed to teach. On the other hand, marriage to men meant sex, pampering and maid service. But the women of the late 19th century began to change history. Of those born between 1860 and 1880, 11 percent never married, the highest rate of unmarried women ever. This was thought to be due to the growing number of women attaining college educations and the male view that college grads made poor homemakers. Leonora Howard was one of those graduates.

The summer of 1872 was an exciting time on the Howard farm, for this year the Board of Governors of the University of Michigan had accepted Leonora as a medical student, to commence formal studies at Ann Arbor, in September 1874. She was one of only 30 women students — there were 275 men. Leonora must first, the governors cautioned, spend two years apprenticed to a qualified physician, and that doctor must act as preceptor, or tutor-sponsor, for her first year at the medical school. Uncle Alpheus, now practising in Grand Rapids, Michigan, would be the perfect candidate.

Women, in fact a number of schoolteachers like Leonora, were entering the medical field at this time, albeit through those more liberal American doors. So far, none could practise in Canada, but England and the United States now boasted quite a select few of these admirable creatures. The battle had been hard fought and even harder won.

Leonora could not really know what she was in for, first because she was, in effect, tucked away in the countryside, and second because the doctors in her family had probably been most encouraging. And although Leonora had attended teacher's college in Syracuse, New York[1] — teaching being the only acceptable occupation for a genteel spinster — she, like most young rural women, had little knowledge of the larger world. The road ahead would certainly be bumpy. But it would be an honest road, fairly and legally obtained, even if, to Leonora's vast disappointment, it would be in another country. One letter to the editor of *The Whig*,* from Donald Maclean in Ann Arbor, stated "Miss Howard has repeatedly expressed to me her regret at having to come to this foreign University in search of the education which she might so much more conveniently have obtained at the Royal College at Kingston within a day's journey of her own home." This was written in response to a letter to the *Adrian Times*, January 21, 1880, describing Leonora as a "Michigan girl."

The first woman to practise medicine in the Dominion of Canada had, in fact, posed as a man. Six years after Leonora had entered this world, Dr. James (Miranda) Stuart Barry, a British Army medical officer, turned up as inspector-general of hospitals for both Upper and Lower Canada. Dr. Barry was the physical and emotional opposite of quiet, feminine Leonora Howard, being all her life aggressively masculine in her behaviour. After obtaining a medical degree from Edinburgh University (dressed as a man), "James" Barry had lived in South Africa, for the most part attempting to rectify the appalling sanitary conditions and even worse nutrition endured by inhabitants of leper colonies. Like Florence Nightingale toiling away in the Crimea, Dr. Barry was aghast at the equally sorry lot of regular army troops, whose mortality rate, due to disease and malnutrition, not active service, was almost double that of civilians. Barry once antagonized so many officials that she was actually arrested and sent home. In this sense Dr. Barry resembled Miss Nightingale, who fought bitter battles

*This was probably the Kingston *Whig*. Letter dated Ann Arbor, January 23, 1880.

against army doctors and governments alike. Florence, the "Lady with the Lamp," had stepped on so many toes that she had almost been tricked into sailing on a ship, supposedly bound for her Crimean hospital, but in fact on its way back to England to get her out of the way.

Dr. Barry had travelled farther and wider than Florence Nightingale (who did not believe that women should be doctors), perhaps because she had the freedom of a male persona. He, or she, left in her turbulent wake some sweeping

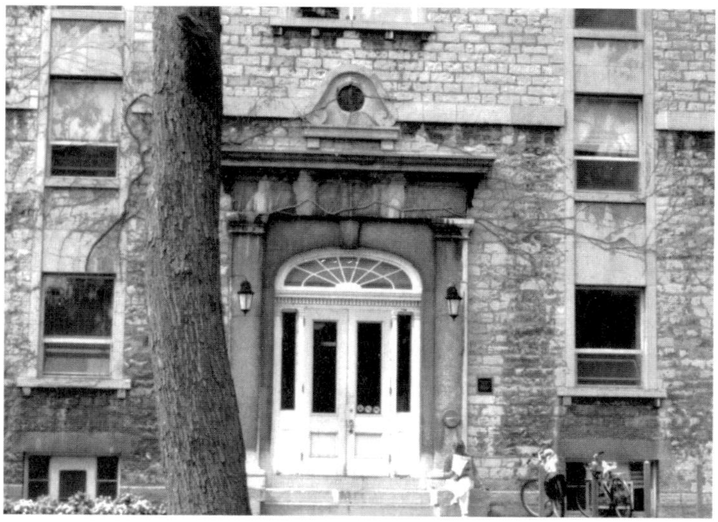

Queen's University, Kingston, Ontario, where Leonora wanted to study

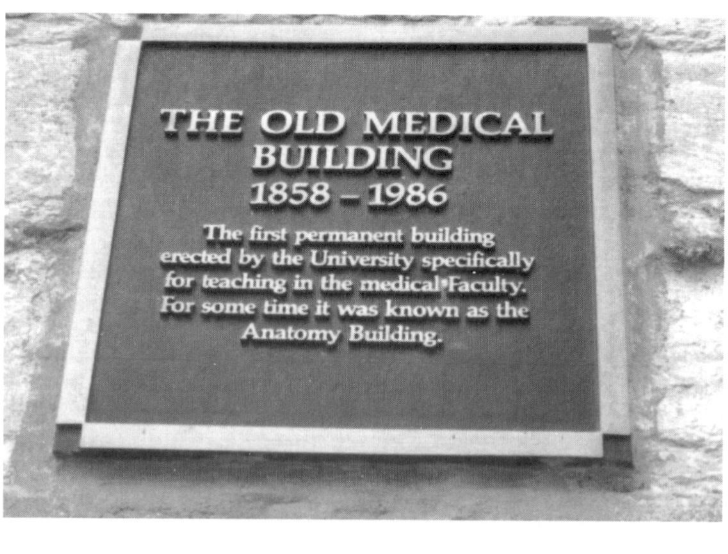
THE OLD MEDICAL
BUILDING
1858 – 1986
The first permanent building
erected by the University specifically
for teaching in the medical Faculty.
For some time it was known as the
Anatomy Building.

reforms in South Africa, Mauritius, Jamaica, St. Helena, Trinidad, Malta, Corfu, Crimea, and eventually, Canada. Her legacy, combined with Miss Nightingale's, had changed the face of the medicine that young Leonora Howard was about to study, forever and for the better.

James Miranda Barry, for all her accomplishments, made enemies throughout her career. Even the dedicated Miss Nightingale, when she met Barry face to face, became "furious," writing:

"He kept me standing in the midst of quite a crowd of soldiers, commissariat servants, camp followers, etc. etc. every one of whom behaved like a gentleman, during the scolding I received, while (she) behaved like a brute. After (she) was dead, I was told (he) was a woman. I should say (she) was the most hardened creature I ever met."

Not to be too hard on Dr. Barry, Florence Nightingale was known to be self-centred, incapable of accepting criticism, and could not herself bear to be denied whatever she asked. Used to the flattery of upper-crust Englishmen, even Queen Victoria's adored consort, Prince Albert, she must have been horrified at such uncavalier treatment. It is interesting that she who was a wizard at manipulating men was repelled by one who was so very "masculine." Perhaps she sensed something the others didn't.

While in Lower Canada (now Quebec), Barry had also decided that both sewage and drainage were inadequate for hygienic purposes, and that pipes should be installed in each army barracks. Hospitals, appalling places in those days, were overcrowded, unventilated, lice-ridden cesspools with unkempt, usually alcoholic "nurses." These harridans earned their few coppers by emptying slop pails and ladling out the bilious-looking boiled "beef." They often made a living through sleeping with whichever patient was in good enough shape. Everyone, therefore, including the "nurses," was at constant odds with bedbugs. Linens in these hospitals told a horror story of their own. Pillows and mattresses of bug-ridden straw became sodden with pus and urine, or crackling-stiff with a former patient's dried blood. Sheets, if available, were not changed for months. Windows were sealed shut, even in the hottest weather.

Little did young Leonora know it, but some 20 years after James Miranda Barry and Florence Nightingale had upset the applecarts with their outlandish demands, she herself, faced with no drainage, no hospitals, not even the semblance of a mattress, would embark on similar reforms that would change the lives of millions. Leonora's methods, however, would be in stark contrast to those practised by Dr. James Miranda Barry.

The first woman to practise medicine in Canada *as a woman* had a number of things in common with Leonora, including a name. Born at Norwich,

Oxford County, Upper Canada in 1831, Dr. Emily Howard Jennings Stowe initially became, like Leonora, a schoolteacher. Refused entry to the University of Toronto, she settled in 1854 for a First Class Teacher's Certificate from what was known as a normal school. Like the future Dr. Howard King, Emily would marry a religious man (Alexander King, Leonora's husband of the distant future, was an ordained minister, while John Stowe was a lay Methodist preacher). But square-jawed, bespectacled Emily was years ahead of her time.

When Leonora was but a child in pinafores, Emily had been teaching at the private Nelles Academy in Upper Canada. There she struck up a great friendship with Dr. William Waggoner Nelles and his brother, Dr. Samuel Sobiestic Nelles, principal of Victoria College in Cobourg, Ontario.[2] Along with her Nelles friendship, dealing with husband John's tuberculosis convinced Emily that she should, and could, become a doctor. Because no Canadian university would accept her she headed for the United States, where the British Dr. Elizabeth Blackwell, the first woman physician, had graduated in 1849 from Geneva (New York) Medical College.

In 1867, the year of Canada's Confederation, Emily returned with her medical degree and began to practise — illegally. Two years later a Canadian Act of Parliament brought in regular licensing laws and appointed a Council of the College of Physicians and Surgeons as sole licensing board for Ontario. Mrs. Emily Stowe, MD, applied for registration and was refused, because the act was carefully worded to bar women from practising medicine, even if they were recognized elsewhere as doctors. One regulation, for example, stipulated that United States graduates must attend one session of lectures at a recognized Ontario medical school and then take a matriculation exam. This was a perfect "out" for the council, because no Ontario medical school would admit women.

Emily Stowe, who was also an ardent suffragette, became increasingly adamant that women be recognized as equal members of society, *and* that she be legally allowed to practise medicine in Canada. Finally, in the early 1870s, the Toronto School of Medicine allowed Mrs. Stowe and Mrs. Jennie Trout, MD, (Women's Medical College of Pennsylvania, 1872), to attend a session of lectures, provided they made "no fuss." There, both Emily and Jennie put up with monstrous abuse, having ghastly items left on their classroom seats, obnoxious sketches displayed on the walls, and being exposed to noisy and "vulgar" medical demonstrations. For all the duo's torment, the Dominion of Canada still refused to grant other women the right to study for and receive full medical degrees.

The University of Michigan's medical school had resolved to accept applications from women just two years prior to Leonora Howard's acceptance. Still, the illustrious Board of Regents did not provide a particularly warm welcome for these aspiring doctors. During the very first women's semester, the medical school faculty formed a committee that submitted a "Memorial on Female Medical Education." At first the professors protested that they held no prejudice against such a practice. They went so far as to say that women were mentally qualified; that their sensibilities and sympathies with the ailing were more pronounced; that many women might prefer devoting their lives to relieving human suffering, and finally, "that a proper sense of delicacy demands that the duties of the accoucher [sic] shall be placed in the hands of women."

All this said, the medical faculty reminded the university's regents that "woman is during a large fraction of each month a quasi-invalid, that her mental and moral manifestations are seriously perturbed at such times ... that child-bearing must incapacitate her during a large part of the period of *utero gestation* ..." and finally, that as child-bearing would be an insuperable obstacle in the way of a female physician, the danger would be that feticide and infanticide, already alarmingly frequent, would become still more so.

So, concluded the committee, medical coeducation would be "an experiment of doubtful utility, and one not calculated to increase the dignity of man, nor the modesty of woman." If the Board of Regents insisted on prevailing in their resolution, the medical men felt that the only workable solution would be to segregate instruction — men in one class — women in another. This, the faculty said, they would be willing to undertake "for suitable compensation" of a whopping $500 extra per professor per annum. Finally, the learned gentlemen suggested a separate female medical college be built either in Ann Arbor or Detroit.[3] The former was the location of choice.

It was to Ann Arbor, then, that Leonora Howard would travel, leaving for the second time in her life the warmth of home, family and the solid little community of Farmersville. Whatever her parents, Peter and Dorothy, thought of this monumental decision is unknown, but Leonora would be safe boarding with Uncle Alpheus. In August 1872, a gleaming trap, perhaps spruced up for the occasion with bright yellow wheels, would carry the this bright young woman to the train station, and on to a wondrous destiny.

Endnotes

1. A newspaper article written in 1935 by Louise Towriss asserts that Leonora was educated as a teacher at the Athens high school (then called the Farmersville grammar school). The mention of New York comes from: Morgan, Henry J. *Types of Canadian Women Past and Present*. Toronto: William Briggs, 1903, p. 186. The author has assumed that the information written during Leonora Howard King's lifetime is more accurate.

2. Victoria College in Cobourg was the first Canadian institution to graduate a woman doctor. That woman was not Emily Stowe, but her daughter, Augusta.
3. McGuigan, Dorothy. *A Dangerous Experiment: 100 Years of Women at the University of Michigan*. Ann Arbor, Michigan: University of Michigan Press, 1970, pp. 35-38.

Chapter two

The lady doctors
1872–1876

Be ye therefore wise as serpents, and harmless as doves.
— Matthew 10:16

Train travel in 1872 was not the most pleasant experience for a woman. "Ladies' cars," in which one could supposedly escape smoking, spitting and unwanted masculine attention, were primarily used in the southern United States rather than in Canada. And even if one were lucky enough to find such a conveyance, husbands or other suitable escorts who accompanied female travellers would ensure that the first two irritants remained unavoidable.

Sustenance was another obstacle entirely. Because this journey was made prior to the advent of the dining car, Leonora probably had to rely upon "Refreshment Saloons," where a train would stop for about 15 minutes, allowing her to disembark, hastily order something to eat, and then run back to the train at an unladylike gallop. One female passenger wrote "If there is any good word in the English language more shamefully misused ... it is the word refreshment ... there could not be a more inappropriate designation for such abominations of desolation." To add insult to injury, once back in the railway car a lady, while attempting to eat, would find herself not only ducking those fearsome brown streams of tobacco juice but just as often pounding out burning cinders that threatened to set her dress, and herself, on fire.[1]

From Kingston, Ontario, Leonora travelled on the brand-new Grand Trunk Railway to Toronto, then down to Niagara Falls, and finally to Windsor, situated just across the river from Detroit. There she was most likely met by Uncle Alpheus. Detroit, even more than Toronto, would have been huge, noisy and bewildering to the rural Miss Howard, but at least there was family to provide some comfort, and the tufted-leather seats of a phaeton carriage were heaven compared with the bone-rattling trains. Perhaps uncle and niece would spend the night here with friends, for Grand Rapids, where Alpheus lived, was almost 160 kilometres away from the peaceful green lawns and shady oaks of Ann Arbor.

The University of Michigan was at the time run by James Burritt Angell, third president of the institution. Angell had taken the position on a the promise of $4,500 a year, plus a house, but most important, he had been given a strong assurance from Acting President Henry Frieze that women entering the school would not prove "troublesome."[2] J.B. Angell was an ambitious man with connections that reached as far as the White House. These connections would eventually land him the post of "United States Ambassador, Envoy Extraordinaire, etc. etc." to China. Though neither of them could know it, James Angell would later, in the exotic setting of North China, make a curious and important connection with his former student. At present, though, all assurances by President Frieze aside, it was unlikely that Leonora Howard's mild and pious temperament would prove remotely "troublesome."

To be admitted to the degree of doctor of medicine, Leonora had to "exhibit evidence of having pursued the study of medicine and surgery for the term of three years with some respectable practitioner of medicine (including lecture terms); must have attended two full courses of didactic instruction ... must have been engaged in the study of Practical Anatomy and Practical Chemistry; must be twenty-one years of age; must have submitted to the Faculty a thesis, composed and written by himself" and finally, must pass a stringent examination. The terms of admission to the medical department also stipulated that Leonora present to the faculty "satisfactory evidence of a good moral character," and unless already a matriculant of the university or a graduate of "some respectable college, academy or high school," she would be examined on previous education and fitness for "entering upon and appreciating the technical study of medicine."

Evidently Leonora's morals were beyond reproach, and she had already attended college in New York State. Now that she was a "Michigan resident" in Uncle Alpheus' house, her entrance fees, payable in advance, were $10. Non-residents paid $25. Her annual dues would be $15, compared with $20 for non-residents. The graduation fee "For all alike" would be $5. Because neither dormitories nor commons were available, woman students had to obtain board in the homes of private families for "from three to five dollars per week." Clubs were also formed, in which board ranged from "one dollar and a half to two dollars and a half per week." Room rent in these clubs varied from 75 cents to $2 weekly. This sounds quite reasonable until reading the following caveat: "The annual expenses for students in the Academic Department for the last few years, including clothing and incidentals, have been, on the average, about $370. The expenses of Law and Medical students are from $150 to $200 per term of six months." Medical school was not for the impoverished.[3]

To be frank, Leonora and her fellow students may, in fact, have benefited enormously by being segregated from some of their sometimes abusive male colleagues. Working with other women alone, at that period in history, produced an astounding number of strong-minded, highly-skilled physicians who might otherwise have buckled under the constant and hostile pressure brought to bear in mixed classes. The men, unfortunately, still took vicious delight in lording it over these "mere slips of girls." But with segregated medical schools, there would be a far more healthy competition and, probably, much better cooperation. It is a fact that Leonora and her female colleagues would not even compete with their own sisters, real nurses who were only just beginning to emerge in England. For by the time Leonora entered the university, Florence Nightingale had introduced the novel idea of dedicated, morally upright, uniformed, *trained* nurses. Even though Leonora would not, in North America at least, work with this new "sisterhood," the first nurses would start their studies in 1873 at the Bellevue Nursing School in New York. They would not be recognizable, with cap and uniform, for three more years.

Leonora's way in Ann Arbor had been paved by Amanda Sanford of Auburn, New York, the first woman to earn her medical degree at the University of Michigan. Unlike some of her male colleagues, Amanda had already received her first degree — at the Female Medical College in Philadelphia. She had also interned for a year at the New England Hospital for Women and Children in Boston. Amanda Sanford remained dissatisfied with her knowledge and, determined to have the best medical education available, opted for further studies at the University of Michigan's medical department, considered by many the best in the country. Dr. Sanford, a handsome woman with large, friendly eyes and an intelligent face, graduated with honours in 1871. She walked up to receive her degree at the university chapel through hoots, jeers, and showers of abusive notes from her "gentleman" colleagues.[4]

But Amanda, indeed Leonora, had made the right choice: the facilities of the university were indeed impressive. The main building consisted of two vast stone structures, one four and the other three storeys high, graced at the entrance by four impressive Doric columns. The university's *Medical Announcement* proudly noted that "The apparatus in the department of chemistry and chemical physics, is probably unsurpassed, if indeed it be equaled [sic] by that of any medical college in the country." Here, Leonora could walk through museums, gazing at a "valuable collection of bones ... models in wax, papier mache and plaster of various portions of the body, illustrating morbid growths, skin diseases, etc., preparations in the comparative embryology, neurology and craniology of the vertebrata; human embryology and anatomy and pathology of the diseases of women, etc." She would also see the university's "collection of monstrosities, both single and double, of man and the lower animals" that was written up as being full and valuable.

The Materia Medica department boasted a "very complete suit of crude organic medicinal substances ... imported from Paris, put up in beautiful glass-covered half gallon jars ... ." On top of all this, Leonora had free access to general botanical, zoological and geological cabinets containing 150,000 specimens. The general library, a student's dream, contained about 23,000 volumes, of which 1,600 were medical works. The chemical laboratory, the only area in which Leonora would study alongside men, occupied some 15,000 square feet, containing 175 tables, "each being supplied with gas and water, and all the apparatus necessary ... ."

With the absolute exception of Dr. James Miranda Barry, the women doctors of the 19th century tended to concentrate on female diseases, particularly those associated with pregnancy and childbirth. But first, the basics. After a two-year apprenticeship with Uncle Alpheus, Leonora spent her first year studying elementary branches of Chemistry, Anatomy, Physiology and Materia Medica. The next year was taken up with a thorough study of "the more advanced branches of Pathology and the Practice of Medicine, of Surgery, of Midwifery and the diseases of women and children, and the specialty of diseases of the eye and ear." An optional third year, which Leonora Howard did not seem to have taken, was suggested, though not mandatory, for a careful review of these latter branches, and to clinical study in the hospital.

Back in 1871, Leonora learned, Amanda Sanford had written her thesis on *Eclampsia Puerperalis*, a dread condition in pregnancy that causes convulsions and often the death of mother and baby. Half of all women afflicted died of this terrible condition. But although Dr. Sanford had devoured enormous quantities of literature in English, German and French, the best treatment she could come up with was "hot vinegar water on the feet, mustard fomentations on the chest, cupping and drawing blood, chloroform to ease the convulsions, and a cork between the teeth to prevent tongue-biting." The medical knowledge of women's problems in the 19th century was, though improving in leaps and bounds, sketchy at best.

"Cupping" and "bleeding," those two ineffective and often dangerous practices, had been used for almost a century. Through the advice of the influential

Benjamin Rush, Professor of the Institutes of Medicine at the University of Pennsylvania (1791 onward), and physician to the Pennsylvania Hospital from 1783 to 1813, thousands of students and professors continued, even in the 1870s, to attach leeches to human skin. Rush, who had a fantastic imagination, convinced many that Black people were that colour due to a form of leprosy; that yellow fever was caused by "noxious miasmas"; that tobacco caused madness and tuberculosis (which latter could be cured by vigorous horseback-riding, opium, or eating meat, along with the ubiquitous bleeding and purging); and that blistering the skin and "puking" would relieve nervous constriction of blood vessels caused by an accumulation of poisons from the disease state. It was little wonder that initially the sick and diseased tried every patent medicine on the market, rather than consult a doctor.

Before 1840, Leonora's grandfather and his colleagues had as a matter of course performed surgery without anaesthetic. Some doctors, more butchers than physicians, went so far as to say "the abolishment of pain in surgery is a chimera ... absurd to go on seeking it ... knife and pain are two words in surgery that must be forever associated in the consciousness of the patients." Happily, nitrous oxide, or laughing gas, first a form of entertainment at parties and exhibitions, began to be used by dentists in 1844. Then ether was introduced, amidst a storm of religious protests, in 1846. Chloroform, favoured by European and Civil War surgeons, made its entrance in 1848. Opium and morphine, courtesy of Britain's tragic trade in far-off China, were also first used extensively during the American Civil War. Morphine, or morphia, could now be found on the dry-goods shelf as "Winslow's Baby Syrup" and "Kopp's Baby Friend" — a temporary mother's friend indeed, but often used with disastrous, lifelong addictive results. Pure opium was used as a mild pain killer and sedative throughout the century.[1] Sold openly in drugstores as laudanum, this viscous sap of the pretty oriental poppy was a favourite with frustrated housewives and well-to-do ladies who had "attacks of nerves." Other bored ladies would stay tiddly most of the time, courtesy of Lydia Pinkham's famous and remarkably popular tonic.

While washing one's hands was de rigeur by this time, Leonora Howard would practise without antiseptics well into the 1880s. Carbolic acid, discovered and strongly recommended as a disinfectant by Benjamin Lister, was looked upon with suspicion in North America. Dr. Samuel Gross, professor of surgery in Philadelphia, wrote in an 1876 medical review that "Little if any faith is placed by any enlightened surgeon ... in the so-called carbolic acid treatment of Professor Lister." As a result of this distrust, millions of people around the world, many of them women in childbirth, continued to die tragically of blood poisoning.

Along with septicemia, the major complaints she dealt with, even in Michigan, were ague (malaria), cholera, consumption (tuberculosis), quinsy (acute tonsillitis), dyspepsia (indigestion, which might also be ulcers or stomach cancer), diarrhea, from which many people died, black vomit (yellow fever), and that age-old complaint, rheumatism. Malaria was not so much killing as debilitating, and so prevalent in North America that one man wrote that to have the ague was so common that the patient could hardly claim the privilege of sickness.

Asiatic cholera, on the other hand, filled the populace with dread, for once you had it, you might not live to see the next day — and of particular horror was the thought of swelling into a blackened, putrefied mass that was so bloated it would not even fit into a coffin for a decent burial. Cholera continued to break out in North America throughout the century. In 1873, while Leonora was apprenticed to Uncle Alpheus, a North American pandemic claimed thousands of lives. There was really nothing the doctors could do except administer clean water. Hospitals, where the already sick would succumb at the first exposure to dysentery, for example, were closed to the dying. Caused in the main by contaminated water and in some cases contaminated food, cholera would run its murderous course in the cooler climes of Canada and the United States until the bacillus, diluted as it passed from person to person, became too weak to do much harm. In China, where Leonora would eventually practise, the habitual use of "night soil" or human feces for fertilizer would produce epidemics well into the next century. But the Chinese knew one thing Westerners didn't: for the most part they boiled every drop of water they drank.

The American children that Leonora Howard would treat as an intern faced the usual diseases of polio, diphtheria, whooping cough, scarlet fever, measles, mumps and chicken pox, as well as tuberculosis, which was a major scourge. In fact, graveyards across the land testified that infants and children suffered a pathetically high death rate throughout the 19th century. It was only in 1882 that Robert Koch would discover the tubercle bacillus. Two years later he would isolate the cholera bacterium, but little would be done about it in the inner cities. A vaccine for measles, which yearly killed millions of children around the world, would not be found for almost 70 years.

Leonora Howard and her colleagues might, in those years, hear that tuberculosis was caused by wearing party or summer dress with bare arms and necks and, for the little ones, short skirts. Treatments for this and other diseases were often fatal, if not severely debilitating. The younger medical students may by then have balked at prescribing the drug calomel, as this highly popular potion was beginning prove equally highly toxic. But if Leonora did not prescribe calomel, it is more certain that she was a strong believer in the universal purge of castor oil taken (to disguise the taste) with blackstrap molasses.

Perhaps to her initial shock, the virginal Miss Howard would also find that contraception was widely practised throughout the continent, and abortion was so common (although by now illegal or left up to the doctor's discretion in a number of places) that courts dealt with it leniently, if at all. Childbirth, of course, didn't bother one a whit, especially having grown up on a farm! But contraception and abortion were never discussed with spinsters, who supposedly had no knowledge of the human sexual act. Back in 1800, an American married couple had produced an average of slightly more than seven children, many of whom would die at birth or before puberty. By 1850, that figure had dropped to 5.42. When Leonora entered medical school, it was approaching 4.24 children per household. Church socials were not the only thing discussed over tea in the parlour.

There were a number of reasons for avoiding pregnancy. It wasn't only that constant childbearing wore most women out by age 30. Many bright young housewives strenuously resisted giving up their girlhood by being saddled with one child a year, losing, in turn, their figures, their beauty, and their physical strength. Those graveyards with the little headstones were also full of larger memorials to sisters and mothers who had either exhausted their childbearing capacity or died when a midwife or surgeon with filthy hands cut or sewed their vulnerable areas. Therefore young women in the know used items such as the "female syringe," a not-so-successful but better-than-nothing option. Although harmless in itself, this device was often sold with chemicals such as alum or sulphates of zinc or iron, to ensure that a husband's contributions went no farther than the hallway. Sponges, attached to a thread, were another not-very-effective method and were often a cause of terrible infection.

Another device commonly used was the pessary, sold in 100 different varieties, ostensibly for the purpose of correcting a prolapsed uterus. Informed women knew its real intent, as one lady wrote to her newlywed friend ." ... the thing we (use) (when I say we I mean us girls) ... hasn't always been *sure* ... but that was our own carelessness ... They are called Pessaire or female preventive if you don't want to ask for a pisser just ask for a female preventive. They cost one dollar ... ."[5]

When Leonora Howard began her formal medical education, she moved to "diggings" at Ann Arbor's peaceful, tree-shaded campus. At just about this time, Canadian Dr. Jennie Trout was finally registered to practise in her own country — the first woman to practise legally in Canada. Her friend, the older, more vociferous Emily Stowe, would not be licensed by the College of

Physicians and Surgeons for another five years. It has been suggested that there are two possible explanations for Emily's late entrance onto the professional scene. The first is that she flatly refused to take an examination, which was partly oral, feeling (probably correctly), that the all-male audience would be hostile to someone who had openly been at war with them for more than 10 years. The second explanation is that Emily had now begun the notorious Toronto Women's Literary Club, which was actually Canada's first suffragette society.

Registered with the college on May 13, 1875, the very same year she graduated in Pennsylvania, Dr. Jennie Kidd Trout was quiet and retiring in comparison to the embattled Emily. Like the gentle, dedicated Leonora Howard, Jennie disliked publicity, although she was well recognized in contemporary records. In addition to her retiring nature, Jennie was frail and, like Florence Nightingale, given to periods of "nervous bodily ailments." She opened an "Electro-Therapeutic Institute" in Toronto and believed that had it not been for her exposure to electrotherapeutics (presumably electroshock therapy), then highly regarded and apparently effective for Jennie, she might never have become a doctor. In 1877, the year Leonora Howard graduated in Michigan, Jennie was written up in a book on the "Notabilities of Toronto." She would go on to become "Benefactor" and "Distinguished Friend" to the newly formed Kingston Women's Medical College, the first of its kind in Canada.

In the beginning, Emily Stowe had given Jennie Trout much encouragement and the two became fast friends. A serious rift may have occurred when Jennie decided to take, and subsequently pass creditably, that dreaded oral examination. Jennie, being like Leonora much more of a "lady," was accepted by the male examiners. The more combative Emily Stowe was left in the wings. Three years after Leonora herself had graduated from the University of Michigan, Augusta Stowe, Emily's daughter, sat the matriculation exam at the Canadian College. She would become the first woman to obtain a Canadian medical degree, and did so one year before her own mother finally received her licence.

During the apprentice years with Uncle Alpheus at Grand Rapids, Leonora had worked as a type of intern, both at local hospitals and at the university's "College Clinics." She observed medical, surgical and ophthalmic patients being examined, prescribed for and, when necessary, operated upon before the class. Because the service was free for the patients, "large numbers of chronic cases, from this and neighboring States, [had] availed themselves of these privileges." Besides the clinics, the regents had, some years past, set apart one of the buildings as a hospital, but finding it inadequate, the state legislature had been asked for and granted a "generous grant (to which a large amount has been added by the city of Ann Arbor)" to erect and furnish a new hospital. Here, Leonora could practise in two shining new pavilions with 5-metre-high ceilings, "amply provided with every appointment of a first-class hospital — baths, water closets, heating and ventilating apparatus, lounging and reception rooms for patients, etc." A few private rooms were provided for those patients willing to pay. Here, a special course of instruction in physical diagnosis was given, for which Leonora would pay an extra fee of $5.[6]

Leonora, most probably by now almost painfully thin, was said to be "poor," and "denied herself many of the comforts of life rather than make her wants known." It is almost certain that had her family members known of this distressing situation, they would have come to the rescue, but perhaps Leonora's pride prevented any request for help. This genteel poverty, the universal plight of the medical student, finally came "to the light and [her wants] were gladly supplied by the good ladies" of Ann Arbor.[7] These ladies of the Methodist Episcopal Church, while happy to help out the less fortunate, had a definite purpose in helping the aspiring doctor. As for Leonora, one cannot be certain if one night, poring over her books by the dim light of a kerosene lamp, she had any vision of a "mission" in other lands. What is certain, though, is that by this time, the American Methodist Episcopal women had formed a strong and vocal group throughout the United States. This powerful organization was known as the Woman's Foreign Missionary Society (WFMS).

Endnotes

1. McCutcheon, Marc. *Everyday Life in the 1800s*. Cincinnati, Ohio: Writer's Digest Books, 1993, p. 70.
2. McGuigan, Dorothy. *A Dangerous Experiment: 100 Years of Women at the University of Michigan*. Ann Arbor, Michigan: University of Michigan Press, 1970, pp. 35-38.
3. University of Michigan. *Annual Announcement, 1875-76*. Ann Arbor, Michigan: Department of Medicine and Surgery, University of Michigan, 1876, pp. 3-11.
4. McGuigan, *A Dangerous Experiment*, pp. 35-38.
5. McCutcheon, *Everyday Life in the 1880s*, pp. 165-171.
6. *University of Michigan, Annual Announcement*, pp. 3-11.
7. Letter to the editor. *Adrian Times* [Michigan] (January 21, 1880).

Chapter three

The call
1877

Go ye into all the world, and preach the gospel to every creature.
— Mark 16:15

Leonora had applied to the WFMS in 1875, while she was still at university. At the annual meeting of the Northwestern Branch, based in Chicago, an earnest request had come up from the missionaries in the foreign field, for lady physicians. This request, reported the branch, brought the subject of medical education of their missionaries into prominence. It was obvious that Leonora Howard was, three quarters of the way through her medical studies, an ideal candidate to fit the WFMS bill. Those kind ladies of Ann Arbor, working for the Northwestern Branch, suggested she be given a student loan in return for her "adoption" by the society.

A few months previous, the Northwestern Branch had decided to refer the matter of assistance in acquiring a medical education to a committee, thereafter called the WFMS Medical Educational Committee. At its third quarterly meeting for 1875–1876, Leonora Howard's credentials were acted upon favorably, and she was duly adopted by the Medical Educational Committee, February 29, 1876. The Chicago Recording Secretary noted, for some reason, that Leonora came from a place called "Lyn, Ontario" instead of Farmersville, and that her father, rather than her uncle, was a physician. Nonetheless, in May 1876 the General Executive Committee of the WFMS "*Resolved*, That the testimonials of Miss Leonora Howard, MD, for general scholarship and medical knowledge, and also for Christian character, are entirely satisfactory, and that we recommend her acceptance by the committee."

The world missionary enterprise was enormously influential in Victorian society, in that women played almost as large a role as men. This was due because women in most "heathen" countries — the South Seas being a vivid exception — were confined in purdah, or harems, and the only way they could be reached was through the ministrations of other women. For that reason alone, the mission boards began to hire women doctors.

In 1876, the year Leonora graduated with her medical degree, there was only one woman doctor in China.[1] The overseas mission, where American Dr. Lucinda Coombs toiled, was one of the few places where Leonora could find work *and* be welcomed by both her male and female contemporaries. In order to enter the foreign missionary field, however, Leonora would continue to work with Americans, because the official Canadian presence in China would not begin until 1892.*

While she was in Canada, it is likely that Leonora had been influenced by missionaries Dr. Virgil Hart and his wife Addie Galiland Hart, who were members of the Methodist church at Soperton. Addie had been the first Canadian woman missionary in China. In 1865, Virgil, an American, had taken his wife on a field trip to China. Virgil Hart became ill in 1888, and Addie returned with him to Burlington, Ontario. Within a year or so, however, dedicated and energetic Addie would persuade her husband to start up yet another China mission. Leonora's hometown of Farmersville became, for Addie, a busy recruiting ground indeed. Two members of Dr. Hart's new mission, Dr. Omar Kilborn and the Rev. George Hartwell, were also from that little Methodist church. In 1891, nine Canadians in all would set out on the Empress of China, the first ship of the exalted Canadian Pacific "Empress" line.[2]

Like Addie Hart, nearly all missionary women had been preachers' wives, at least prior to the American Civil War. This had presented a bit of a problem, as inevitably, the demands of husband, children, even servants, conflicted with evangelical work. The overwrought, lonely wives finally balked, and as a result of this triple workload, married women in the field were the first to request the services of their single sisters. Although Leonora Howard may have leapt at the chance to travel, she may not have known that the spinster missionary would remain for decades a second-class citizen.

Single women served, often in combination with the preachers' wives, as teacher, nurse, or tract distributor, but lacking ordination they could not administer sacraments or fulfil the ministerial functions of their male counterparts. The prejudice against them was blatant: first, they had to board with married couples rather than occupy their own "diggings," and second, they

*Although the Hart excursion was the first official Canadian presence in China, Jonathan Goforth, the first Canadian evangelist, had, in fact, arrived in China four years previously. Owing to language and other difficulties, he and his wife would not be able to start their mission in Honan Province until the 1890s.

were paid only half as much as the men. Other reasons for "home board" prejudice against spinsters were the opportunity for rumour and criticism that their presence afforded the extremely prudish Chinese, and many women's willingness to leap into marriage with bachelors or widowers in the field, regardless of denominational affiliation.

This latter behaviour became a real bone of contention with the WFMS, for once a woman married, she automatically left her own society for that of her husband's. Hence the organization that sent Leonora out to China would suffer considerable loss in terms of financial investment and valuable experience, including linguistic skills, should she decide to marry. Still China, with particularly rigid gender roles, was the ideal spot to set up a vast enterprise of "Women's work," entailing proselytizing and building schools, orphanages and hospitals for the women and children, because it was impossible for men to gain access to the one-half of the Chinese population that was most pliable, and therefore easiest to convert.

"Women's work" performed in the American Civil War had convinced even diehard male-dominated missionary boards that the ladies had something very special to offer. Apart from an obvious eagerness to do volunteer work, their fundraising ability was astounding. In fact, women's energies over the next 50 years would far surpass those expended by men. Bored with a return to the drudgery of Victorian housewifery, middle-class women, given the new and exciting cause of world evangelism, were most decidedly on the move. In 1869, the Woman's Board of Missions of the Congregational Church, the first denominational board in the United States was founded, and later that same year, the Methodist WFMS sprang up in competition. The real competition, however, was still from the male-dominated General (Missionary) Board, but this was felt more severely in the American South, where opposition to women's work was traditionally greater than in the North. In British Canada, women's overseas missionary work was simply vetoed by the churches.

When Leonora joined the WFMS, the Methodists were the largest single Protestant denomination in the United States, with some 4.7 million members, 25,000 churches and 16,500 pastors. They had also been in China since 1847. China remained, aside from India, the largest Methodist missionary field, accounting for a third of that organization's world force and $4.5 million in property. To support this vast enterprise, American Methodists contributed about half a million dollars a year for missionary upkeep and work, to which sum was added the support of unmarried women missionaries like Leonora, pledged separately by the WFMS.[3]

Leonora was not swept into these ladies' arms just because she was a nice person. The "Rules Governing the Selection and Employment of Missionaries" were quite clear about the type of woman the society wanted. In order to gain assistance, and to be accepted as a missionary, the 24-year-old medical student had, among other things, to answer the following Questions to Applicants:

1. Do you trust that you are inwardly moved by the Holy Ghost to take upon you the work of a foreign missionary?
2. Do you desire and intend to make this your life work, and are you willing to labor in any field?
3. Have you an experimental knowledge of salvation through the atonement of Jesus Christ our Lord? (They probably meant "experiential.")

The religious questions went on but then, more practically,

6. Have you a thorough English education?
7. Have you studied Latin or any modern language, what proficiency have you made, and do you readily acquire the same?
8. In what schools have you taught, and with what success?
9. Have you knowledge of music, either vocal or instrumental?
10. What is the condition of your health?
11. Have you ever been married? If so, is your husband living?
12. Will you answer by *testimonials* to each of these questions?"

Then, the good ladies of the WFMS were equally bound by their own selection rules, which were, in part, to determine that:

1. A missionary candidate must believe herself divinely called to the work of a foreign missionary, and assert her belief that she is actuated only by a desire to work in accordance with God's will.
2. She must here indicate her ability to work in a foreign field by Christian usefulness at home.
3. She must declare her intention to make foreign missionary work the service of her effective years, and agree to give at least five of these years of continuous service, as a single woman ... unless prevented by ill health; she must also assert her willingness to labor in any field, though her preference is always to be taken into account.

In addition to requiring "satisfactory testimonials in regard to scholarship," the WFMS felt that both teaching experience and medical/nursing knowledge were very desirable commodities. With both requisites neatly tucked under her belt, Miss Leonora Howard, soon to be MD, was just what the society wanted. Leonora was also just the right age — a candidate could not be "less than twenty-two years, nor more than thirty." The reasons for this stipulation were fairly basic: a very young woman might not possess the appropriate academic credentials; she might easily change her mind or even worse, become affianced at the last minute; and she might not realize the long-term ramifications of her decision. Women over 30 were a risk, first because their stamina, a prerequisite for field work, might not match that of their younger sisters, and second because "older" women could become a nuisance by questioning and even rebelling against home-board policy decisions.

Leonora also had to be able to balance books, because the WFMS was extremely serious about their financial state at all times. Item six of the rules read "Financial and executive ability, and power of adaptation to circumstances, are essential qualifications."

The women of the WFMS were out to prove to the men of the General Board that they indeed knew how to run a business. The society was, in fact, the group most responsible for underpaying single women in the field, reasoning, perhaps, that the extra money could be better spent on the schools and hospitals they intended to set up. Every missionary candidate was required to sign a contract stating, "I agree to conform to the above requirements and conditions while in the employ ..., and failing in this, to refund the amount of outfit and passage money."

Before being granted her student loan, Leonora was required to read and agree to the WFMS *Instructions to Missionaries*, which stated, among other items, that while in the field she would be expected to attend annual meetings and conferences; report quarterly to her superintendent; send annual and quarterly reports to the corresponding secretary; prepare, along with missionary wives, financial estimates for the ensuing years; incur no expense without prior approval by the board; credit to the society all donations received and report said donations annually; and devote her "entire time and attention" to her legitimate work, "as all temporal necessities will be provided for by the Society." Daunting as all this may have seemed, Miss Leonora Howard signed on the dotted line and in return received $120 to finish her studies at the University of Michigan.

In June 1876, Dr. Howard graduated "with honor" from Ann Arbor. Although she presumably returned home for a much-needed rest, she would shortly return to the United States, there to collect "$200 for personal outfit ... $100 for the furnishings of the Home." The latter, she was reminded, would remain the property of the WFMS.[4] Leonora's salary, which would have to pay for food, lodging, clothing and travel expenses in the field, would be $350 yearly.

Thus the WFMS appointed Leonora Howard, MD, to Peking, China, there to work in association with Dr. Lucinda Coombs. It seems likely, in retrospect, that Leonora had chosen China because of her church connection with Addie Hart, and in this case she was luckier than poor Lucinda. Before Lucinda had even attended medical school, she had resolved to offer herself for service in India. Instead she had bowed to the ladies of the WFMS in their decision to send her to China, saying wistfully "I had hoped to go to India, but it is all the same. It is work for the Master, and the souls of the Chinese women are as dear to him as the souls of the women of India."[5]

When Leonora arrived on the scene, the Methodists were a large, though not the predominant, missionary force in China. In 1877, there was more than enough of China for all the various churches and their sometimes eccentric offshoots. The geographical divvying up among religious groups from many countries came to be known as "conversion rights." There was, as a result of this division of conversion territories, little overlap in the field, but the Roman Catholics, who had been there for centuries, sometimes established rival missions, reported by the Protestants as drawing converts by offering "better soup," or other appropriate inducements. It was a community of odd fellows: in bad times, all the overseas missions pulled together, but in good, there was a healthy, sometimes quite un-Christian rivalry in pulling in the converts. Women as well as men exuberantly entered the fray by competing for higher conversion figures, in the hope of raising some extra cash for God's work.

The WFMS itself was part of an extensive interlocking system, which lent credibility to the Methodist belief that it, outside of the Roman Church, was the most highly organized church body in the world. To mediate among the many concerns competing for attention and funds, the main Methodist Board created a World Service Commission as a central receiving and disbursing agency for foreign missions, home missions, the Epworth League for Young People, the American Bible Society, the Temperance Society, and other special church responsibilities. Each year the commission set a quota for each board to ensure that fundraising did not become the kind of game that "would pit an antirum group against a North China bishop, which was by no means an unknown circumstance."[6]

While there was considerable variation in the background of male missionaries, the young woman offering her services was a far more predictable type. Like Leonora, she was usually from a large rural family — in fact more than a quarter of the fathers of female volunteers on the American board were, like Peter Howard, farmers.[7] Like Leonora, the typical field missionary had worked her way through college by teaching intermittently. And finally, like Leonora, many had passed the age at which it was reasonable to expect a marriage proposal.

Educated women were not in 1870 considered very feminine — professional women were looked upon as downright eccentrics. Also into the femininity issue came the question of a woman's right to be independent, anathema in most middle-class families. Because Leonora and the other farmer's daughters had grown up with much more freedom than had their urban sisters, the tethers, not to mention the corsets of adulthood, might have been difficult to accept. Therefore, if these independent young spirits could get away from obligations to an ailing mother or to younger siblings, they would very probably find the foreign field an exciting and rewarding outlet.

Although some young women sprang into the missionary field with surprising zeal, there existed for most a very serious decision. Depending on the way one looked at it, there was the distinct drawback of homesickness and the seductiveness of autonomy. Coupled with the former would be the loneliness of watching the comfortable existence of a married couple, and perhaps worse, the closeness of mother and children with whom the spinster must board. In addition, the prospects of joining such homey ranks were not high: to a far greater extent than her male counterparts, Dr. Leonora Howard would surrender herself to the single life in an environment where eligible members of the opposite sex were rare indeed.

On the positive side, missionary field work offered her an opportunity to escape the stigma of unladylike professionalism that she would endure at home. There may have been other very personal reasons for Leonora's decision, but it seems, in retrospect, unlikely that she was part of the handful of medical workers who felt an almost nun-like surrender to God's work. To illustrate, one impressionable young China candidate expressed her "desire to live a holy life and to help others to do the same ... and the fact that what once were pleasures and joys to me in the world are not so now."[8]

The male attitude toward women doctors was that while they would never employ female physicians at home, they felt that giving the ladies medical training for work on mission grounds was quite rational.[9] It was, for the men of the mission boards, the devil and the deep blue sea: they frankly had no choice but to hire women if they wanted to obtain universal conversion. Some of the more romantically inclined went to extremes in protesting their support of women. One gentleman almost deified these "Lady Doctors" as "not mere pretentious adventurers, but regular, well-educated physicians, actuated by the purest motive, immolating themselves upon the altar of humanity in order to lay the foundations for bestowing the blessings of a western medical knowledge upon ... their downtrodden sisters in heathen lands."[10]

But this verbal bouquet aside, few roses were tossed at the women who went overseas. Some 10 years after Leonora had single-handedly established four dispensaries, three hospitals, and a mobile field practice, one Baptist board secretary was still thundering that "women's work in the foreign field must be careful to recognize the headship of man ...We must not allow the major vote of the better sex ... nor the ability ... nor even the exceptional faculty for leadership ... to discredit the natural and predestined headship of man in Missions, as well as in the Church of God: and the head of woman is the man."[11]

Masculine bluster notwithstanding, women remained more active in their support than men. Over the next 20 years, more than 40 percent of the general board's income would emanate directly from the women's boards, and even more funding might be credited to female members if their share of regular church contributions could be calculated. In years to come, a 10-year-old Women's Society of the Free Methodist Church of North America would collect more money in a single four-year period than the male-dominated general board had produced in its entire 32-year existence. Whether it was tapping a cymbal and singing *Bringing in Chinese* to the tune of *Bringing in the Sheaves*, or simple social pressure, a significant aspect of North American women's importance is the fact that as early as 1891, their societies contributed more than twice as much as their British counterparts.[12]

Medical missionary work, while relatively new at this point, was seen, variously, as exemplifying Christ's purely selfless work among the sick and maimed, or more practically, as an almost foolproof channel through which to reach "the heathen." No one is more vulnerable than when ailing, and by now both the American board and the WFMS knew it. After 45 years in China, a formidable, bearded patriarch named Reverend R.H. Graves wrote, quite reasonably, "Here...we have the warrant and the work of the medical missionary — as a physician to heal the suffering body, and as a messenger from God to tell the patient of Jesus." Thus, he added, there were two classes of labourer sent out by Christ: ordained ministers to preach and found churches, and incidentally to employ healing "as an aid in their great work," and those like Leonora Howard who would do the "preliminary work of healing, but are never to forget the immortal soul while caring for the perishing body." In China, he wrote, "we find it especially useful in opening new stations, by overcoming the prejudices of the people and showing the benevolent aspect of Christianity in a way that the simplest may understand."

In April 1877, after delivering a speech to the members of the WFMS in Chicago, Miss Leonora Annetta Howard, MD, boarded a train for San Francisco and sailed to Shanghai. She was 26 years old. The WFMS wrote ecstatically that "Our knowledge of her talents and her Christian character warrant the brightest hopes for her future in medical missionary work."[13] In just two years, Leonora would succeed beyond her sponsors' wildest dreams.

Endnotes

1. Dr. Lucinda L. Coombs arrived in Peking in late August, 1873. Source: Wheeler, Mary Sparkes. *First Decade of the Woman's Foreign Missionary Society of the Methodist Episcopal Church*. New York: Phillips & Hunt; Cincinnati: Walden & Stowe, 1881, pp. 161-163.
2. Austin, Alvin J. *Saving China: Canadian Missionaries in the Middle Kingdom, 1888-1959*. Toronto: University of Toronto Press, 1986, p. 52.
3. Fairbank, John K., ed. *The Missionary Enterprise in China and America*. Cambridge, Mass.: Harvard University Press, 1974, p. 284.
4. *Seventh and Thirteenth Annual Reports of the Woman's Foreign Missionary Society*: "Report of Medical Educational Committee" and "Uniform Readings." 1877, pp. 37-39; 1882, pp. 90-93.
5. Wheeler, *First Decade*, pp. 161-163.
6. Fairbank, *Enterprise*, p. 285.
7. Hunter, Jane. *The Gospel of Gentility - American Women Missionaries in Turn-of-the-Century China*. New Haven: Yale University Press, 1984, p. 29.
8. Fairbank, *Enterprise*, p. 77.
9. Austin, *Saving China*, p. 172.
10. Ibid., p. 172.
11. Hunter, *The Gospel of Gentility*, p. 14.
12. Fairbank, *Enterprise*, p. 83.
13. *Seventh Annual Report of the Northwestern Branch of the Woman's Foreign Missionary Society*. Chicago: 1877, pp. 37-39.

Map of China

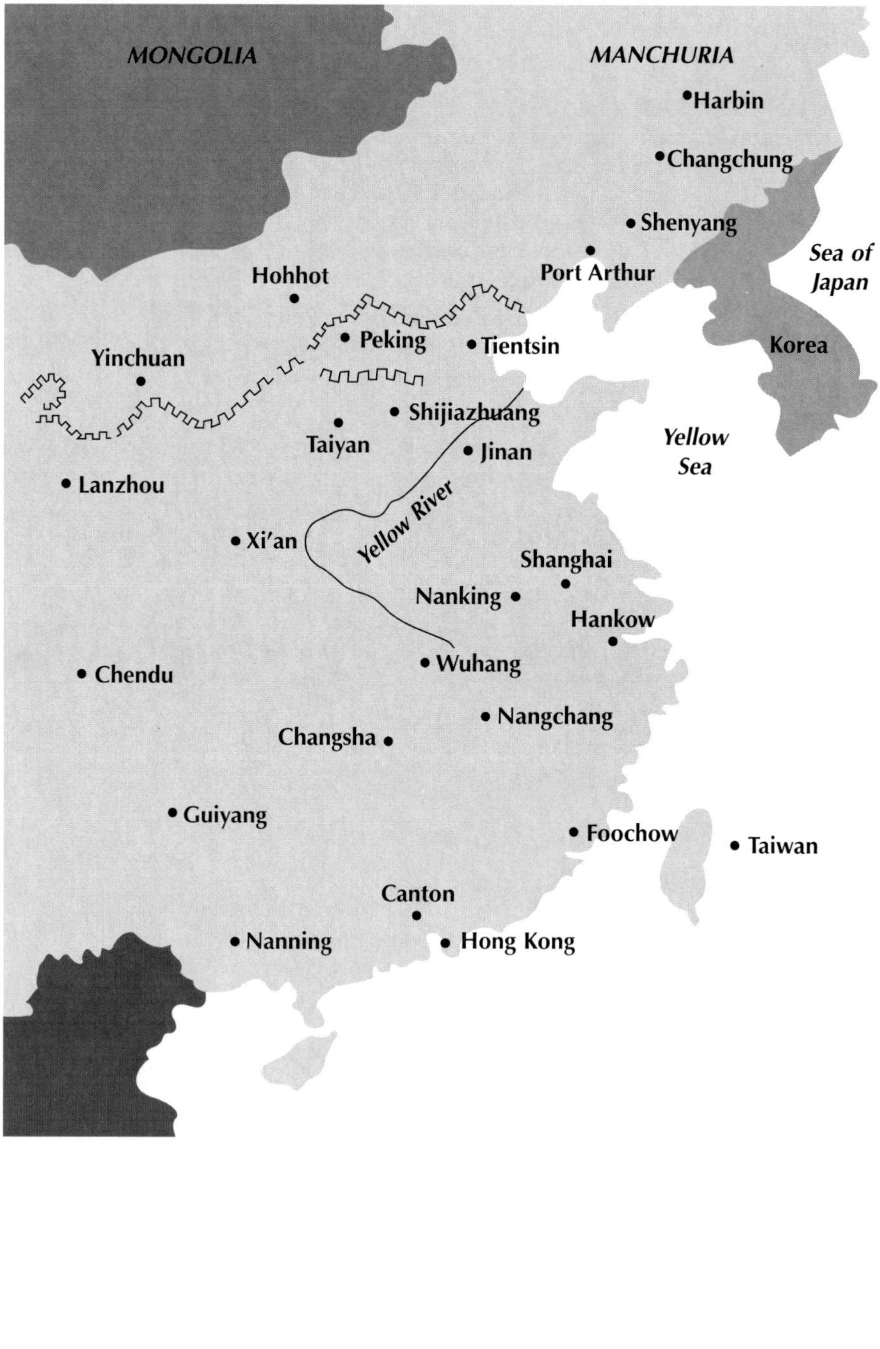
MONGOLIA
MANCHURIA
Harbin
Changchung
Shenyang
Port Arthur
Sea of Japan
Hohhot
Peking
Tientsin
Korea
Yinchuan
Shijiazhuang
Taiyan
Jinan
Yellow Sea
Lanzhou
Yellow River
Xi'an
Shanghai
Nanking
Hankow
Wuhang
Chendu
Nangchang
Changsha
Guiyang
Foochow
Taiwan
Canton
Nanning
Hong Kong

Chapter four

Arrival
1877

Let us not be weary in well doing:
For in due season we shall reap, if we faint not.
— Galatians 6:9

Life on the high seas came as a considerable surprise to the newest missionaries. From San Francisco Leonora would embark on one of America's finest new steamers, probably that well-regarded ship called the *City of Tokio*. Steeled, often eager for privation, many religious workers found themselves comfortably ensconced in first-class cabins, the only concession to the "plain life" being, perhaps, shared accommodation. In between superb ten-course dinners,[1] the men and women of God spent a few days getting to know each other, holding prayer meetings, or reading the tracts they were expected to distribute to "the heathen." Then the fun began, for rest of this three-week crossing was filled with social teas, charades, a game or two of whist for the more daring, and "musicales" performed, if not with professionalism, great amateur gusto.

For the more conservative, the ships would seem excessively luxurious, with the glitter of white-enamelled walls — the latest Victorian fashion — huge mirrors, elegant staircases, and gilding that shone softly in the glow of new "Pintsch" gas lights, introduced to North America just over 10 years past. But on many occasions, there was a darker side to the fine sea voyages. Far below the comfortable salons, below the crystal chandeliers, below the tinkling pianoforte and the spacious cool cabins, hundreds of Chinese coolies rotted and died in their own filth. Returning home from building the white man's railroads, these men had been packed like so many animals into the fetid hold of the ship, then locked in with strong iron grilles "to prevent mutiny."[2] What had once been imagined as a triumphant return to wife and concubine in the Middle Kingdom had been turned into a tragic death camp.

Leonora could not have picked a worse time to travel to North China, for this was the year of the great Yellow River flood. Millions had died and millions more would flock to the cities, gaunt with starvation, ravaged by disease. Bandits roamed the countryside, screaming down on each village to plunder a farmer's little hoard of food. In 1877, a man could convert to Christianity in the morning and sell his daughter that very night, a worthless female being just one more mouth to feed. Perhaps the hardy man in the hold who lived through this nightmare voyage would never find his wife or his concubine. Indeed perhaps his entire village had disappeared in the murderous floods.

Leonora's ship had first taken her to Nagasaki, Japan. At that strange and wonderful city, a change in accommodation was made to an equally well-appointed Japanese steamer that swiftly moved south into warmer climes. Now, just a few hours away from Shanghai, she would see the limpid blue of the Pacific change to the turbid murk of the Yellow Sea. The sea was in fact quite yellow, because every year without fail, tons of red, yellow and grey silt washed down from the hills into the great Yangtze River.* The Yangtze in turn bestowed this dubious gift to the vast salt waters, then the bilious stuff spread out, clouding the water for miles before surrendering at the gates of the Pacific.

Where for days there had been endless, flat horizon with nary a companion ship in sight, Leonora's vessel joined hundreds of fishing boats, junks with their strange brown horizontal sails, paddleboats, single-oared sampans and perhaps a dozen other steamers from ports the world over, all headed for an indefinite brownish haze on the horizon. Leonora's first glimpse of exotic China was two long thin yellow lines that slowly materialized into flat marshland topped with bleak, windswept scrub. No mountains soared in the distance, no graceful temples dotted the landscape — there were no landmarks of any kind. But something was going on, because all of a sudden the noise was deafening. After nothing but the soft whoosh of the ocean and the occasional cry of a gull, here was a sudden, overwhelming cacophony of shouting, clanking, and the nerve-wracking scream of rusty anchor chains. The Japanese steamer had entered Huangpu,† the river of Shanghai.

Leonora had been sick throughout the journey and would suffer from seasickness for the rest of her life. She might well have turned two shades greener as the indescribable "odour of China" assailed her nostrils, but the sight of the great port could make anyone forget their ills. Thousands of dock-workers moved through foreign *hongs*, or warehouses, huge wharves, and building yards.

*The Yangtze is called Changjiang by the Chinese.

†The Huangpu was known to the westerners as the Whangpoo.

Stately American schooners, huge two-storey paddleboats and busy tugs vied with junks large and small, a thousand sampans, and tiny fishing boats. The ship's whistle blew, the engines shuddered, and the Japanese steamer came to rest at Hongkew, the bright new American settlement at Shanghai.

It was hot. It was stifling. It was agony to be dressed in high-laced Balmoral boots, thick lisle stockings, long petticoats layered over a cotton chemise that reached the knee, heavy bustle attached to the waist and a strong black serge skirt to cover the whole. Trying to breathe in that corset-like, tight-fitting boned bodice stretching from waist to upper chest, fastened sternly with 30 small strong buttons must have taken supreme effort. Underneath Leonora's bodice would have been a stiff boiled shirt with high neck that scratched unmercifully in the dense steaming heat. The only sensible item, in fact, would be a broad-brimmed straw travelling hat to protect Leonora's milk-white skin from the merciless, broiling sun.

We must assume that Leonora did not travel alone — indeed she would have been hard-pressed to find her way out of that hellish harbour, let alone journey on to Peking by herself. She and her fellow missionaries would have been met by Methodist Board members at Shanghai harbour, then likely plopped into a *jinricksha*, the first syllable of which had recently been dropped by the Westerners "for convenience." All she could do was hang on for dear life and watch the teeming throngs, a vast human ocean composed of coolies, merchants, dock workers and disreputable-looking sailors on their way to Shanghai's red light district. A torrential rain, typical of the season, may suddenly have obliterated the view and soaked her to the skin.

Shanghai rains stop as suddenly as they begin, almost as if a faucet has been turned off. Magically the crowds and the smells would have diminished in intensity. The air now opened up like some vast exotic flower. The velvet lawns and wide clean boulevards of Shanghai's British "Bund" stretched ahead like some wondrous fairyland. For more than a kilometre Leonora would sway past quietly rich entrances of huge Anglo-Oriental banks, stately hotels, and old established shipping offices.* In the distance, magnificent homes sat back in stately manner, oblivious to the crass commerce of this hugely lucrative port.

Servants of the rich trudged by with wheelbarrows loaded with provisions. A *compradore*, an English-speaking "go-between" for the Westerners might stand, arms folded, by the great carved doors of the Hong Kong and Shanghai

*What came to be known as the "unequal treaties" imposed on China after the Opium Wars of 1840 threw Shanghai open to much foreign traffic, primarily opium. Between 1845 and 1914, western powers seized 4,000 hectares of cultivated land around Shanghai.

Bank. This man would be dressed in rich embroidered silks, as indeed he had a right to be, because the Westerners, except for the missionaries, refused to "lower themselves" to speak Chinese. The multilingual compradores, who took a substantial "squeeze" with each business deal, had become rich beyond their wildest dreams. Then, just around the corner at Bubbling Wells Road, grand open carriages boasted liveried coachmen and well-dressed Western women. The missionaries, bumping along in their rickshaws, would be politely ignored. Leonora would then pass beautiful Huangpu Park, built just 11 years ago. A sign posted at its entrance read: "Chinese and Dogs not admitted."

Leonora could not, with propriety, stay in one of those grand hotels lining the Bund, but the two weeks she would spend in this most Westernized of China's ports would, like the ship she sailed on, be far more comfortable than expected. The young doctor would stay in a spacious Western-style missionary residence house off the main promenade where the huge mansions reigned, but impressive enough in its own middle-class solidity. More than one missionary, expecting screaming hordes of "the heathen," waving things that vaguely resembled scimitars, was confused and somehow disappointed with the distinct Western character of her Shanghai surroundings.

But a week or two's stop at Shanghai was essential for all foreigners travelling on to Peking. The latter, as capital of the Middle Kingdom, was a closed city, and the establishment of foreign-owned stores in Peking was expressly prohibited. Shanghai, however, was a major treaty port where everyday goods were obtained with ease. In addition to seeing to her own needs, Leonora must now consult an extensive shopping list sent home by Peking-based Dr. Lucinda Coombs and her missionary colleagues, Miss Campbell and Miss Porter.[3] An item of paramount importance was good North American butter — a substance sadly lacking in China. Those missionaries who lived in the field always had a cow or two, but homesick urban stomachs demanded that the precious spread be shipped to China by the well-chilled ton.

Ladies' shoes, dresses, bonnets and "unmentionables" were unobtainable, even in Shanghai. Men had better luck. Shanghai's tailors could whip up a masterpiece of tuxedo or riding togs better, more cheaply and faster than their overseas competition. Envious, the Western women would within a few years have their way, and by presenting fashion plates to the master tailors, begown themselves in the latest Paris creations made of the best Shanghai silk. Nanking Road boasted hundreds of stores along its 5-kilometre length. Western crockery, cutlery and exquisite table and bed linens abounded, and glassware was available in every size and shape. Then there was the question of one's bed. More than one foreigner was warned to arrive complete with bedstead, because the brick *k'ang* of the Chinese was far from comforting to large bones accustomed to feather mattresses. For floor covering, "Canton matting" was the preferred material, barring, of course, the arrival of a prized Aubusson rug that took forever to be shipped from home.

Important to missionary and diplomat alike was the issue of light — light by which to dance, to clink champagne glasses, to tuck into velvety prawn bisque and creamy souffles, light by which to tend the sick and the maimed, to mend one's tattered chemise, and to write those endless missionary reports. Until recently the Chinese had used rapeseed (canola) oil to light their dim parlours, but kerosene, with its bright, consistent flame, was fast becoming the fuel of choice for Chinese and foreigner alike. One diplomatic communiqué suggested that an arriving American arm himself with "not less than 20 cases of kerosine [sic] oil at Shanghai" — the best and cheapest assuredly to be found at the American-owned China and Japan Trading Company.[4]

Leonora would also shepherd enormous supplies of items that were unavailable even in Shanghai. The markets far to the north in Peking did offer meats, but after the latest flood one could only find a limited range of vegetables, and a small variety of poor fruit. Soap, candles, tinned goods, flour, starch, vinegar, oil, pepper, raisins, syrup, cheese, and the prized butter not only had to be brought from home but kept from spoiling in the torrid port cities. This shopping on a grand scale was managed with the help of "Old China Hands" and somehow the tons of goods shipped to Asia seemed to reach their destinations with little spoilage. But owing to the isolation imposed by natural disaster such as flooding or the ever-present danger of banditry, self-sufficiency was the order of the day. It was said that the storerooms at the American Legation in Peking carried enough of such articles to stock "a good grocery store" back home.[5] The large Methodist compound where Leonora would live, while hardly needing tins of Beluga caviar, would assuredly have an equal amount of more plebeian stores.

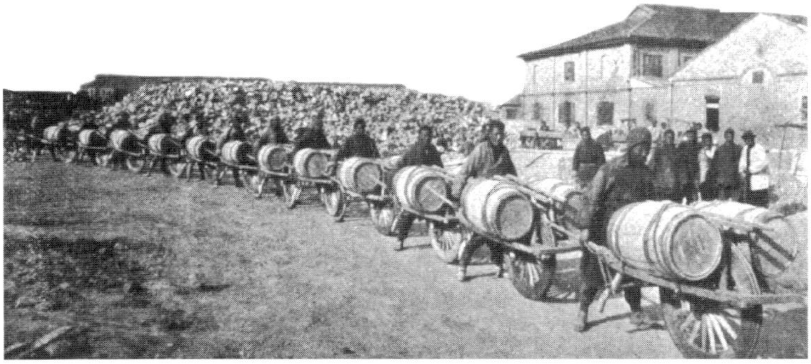

Coolies in Shanghai

It is important to describe Shanghai, even if we shall not visit that city again, for here is the first glimpse of a curiously divided society where the immigrants live far better than the inhabitants. In 1877, Shanghai, like other areas "conceded" in the treaties resulting from the Opium Wars, was divided into two distinct cities. The old city was occupied solely by Chinese, and was seldom, if ever, visited by Westerners. The trading city, with a population of some 200,000, was set firmly within the foreign boundary, subject to foreign municipal laws, and to foreign sanitary regulations. This area retained distinctly Chinese architecture. The cleanliness of the foreign portion's air was due to an expensive but highly successful Westernized sewage system. In addition, water carts kept the dust down in dry weather, and "scavenger's carts" cleaned the streets three times daily. The waterworks supplied an abundance of pure drinking water with a surprisingly high and consistent pressure.

"Concession" was not, in fact, a synonym for settlement. A Chinese concession was a piece of land leased by a foreign government and let, in turn, to Western merchants. The stipulation was that the land would not be sublet to Chinese. A *settlement* was an area within which Westerners could lease land directly from Chinese proprietors.

At the end of the 19th century, Shanghai boasted two telegraph lines to London, a number of daily newspapers, several magazines, and communication with the West at least once a week, courtesy of the mail steamers. Wonderful libraries and the large bookstore of Messrs. Kelly & Walsh catered to those who chose to read, but it was unlikely that the social whirl of winter, combined with the lethargy produced by a humid spring and summer, would encourage much heavy study. Western women were particularly busy socially, because a plethora of servants had reduced household cares to a minimum, and an absence of children, packed home to respectable schools, had added to the ennui experienced by many wives. To the outsider, the frenzied activity was almost frightening: Isabella Bird, adventurer, reported houseboat picnics, shooting excursions, pony races and steeplechase, theatricals, and clubs. There were the Yachting Club, the Golf Club, the Athletic Club, the Lawn Tennis Club. There were the Cricket Club, the Rifle Club, the Boating Club and the Bowling Club. For the higher brow there were the Philharmonic and Photographic societies, the Royal Asiatic Society, and the Fine Art Society. This list, suggested Miss Bird, was just the tip of an exhaustive iceberg.[6]

On the whole, though, merchant, diplomat and missionary would never really meet. Back in 1869, British Lord Clarendon had said "Missionaries require to be protected against themselves, and they are a constant menace to British interests." An American diplomat saw missionaries as "the only barrier between the unhesitating advance of commercial adventure and the not incongruous element of Chinese imbecile corruption," while a British consul told London, "Immense services might be rendered to our commercial interests if only the members of the various missions in China would co-operate with our Consuls in the exploitation of the country."

The missionaries themselves had many of their own activities, but few of the merchant class or diplomatic corps chose to join in. There might be a tip of a hat at Sunday service or a generous donation for an orphanage, for from the earliest days of foreign "occupation" both Protestant and Catholic cathedrals dominated this strange community. Within a few years Leonora would learn about "mission houses" being built in many major centres, the most important being the substantial headquarters of the China Inland Mission, with home for a hundred missionaries, a hospital, goods and business departments, and excellent postal arrangements.

British and American bible societies and the English Religious Tract Society were the most active groups in Shanghai. A great deal of money was made by missionaries who translated "pure and useful" Western literature for the "elevation" of the Chinese. Leonora would meet the women who administered the ample coffers of the Ladies' Benevolent Society for Western widows and children in distress, and the Sailors' Home and Rest, where ladies and gentlemen alike would play and sing at wholesome musical evenings.[7] Shanghai's hospitals, built and run by male missionaries, were segregated, not only between men and women, but most particularly between Westerner and Chinese.

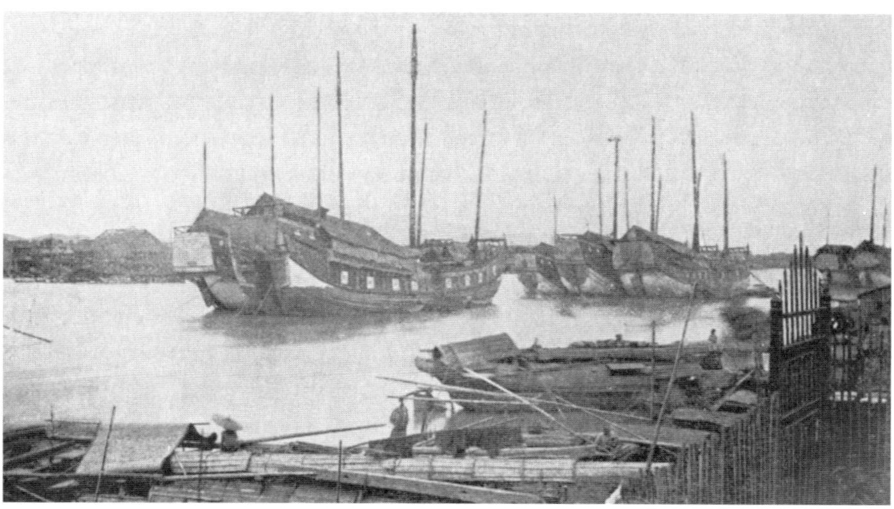

Junks and other boats

The wealthy Chinese who lived in the foreign settlement paid for these advantages through municipal taxes and "feu duty" for their land, which was held in the name of a foreigner. The former, including some mandarins, the compradores and silk merchants, lived under the jurisdiction of the Chinese government, but civil cases in which foreigners were concerned were held in a mixed court. Serious criminal cases reverted to the Chinese Shanghai magistrate. Security was tight, but usually quite unnecessary. Leonora, used primarily to one county reeve who kept law and order, would marvel at elegant Sikh mounted police and a mixed force of Europeans, Sikhs and Chinese patrolling the city day and night.

But there existed another Shanghai, unsavoury and forbidding to the Western mentality. This city, which led its own life according to Chinese custom, had existed long before a 1756 memorandum, drawn up by a Mr. Pigou, which had suggested Shanghai as a desirable trading centre. The industrious Chinese had, centuries before, hit upon exactly the same idea, for Shanghai, the sole outlet of the province of Sze Chuan, was connected by waterways with the great cities of Hangchow and Soochow, far-off Tientsin and with the Great Capital of Peking.

Chinese Shanghai was protected by a high wall that ran about six kilometres in circumference. It is unlikely that Leonora, protected in the artificial atmosphere of the foreign settlement, would have seen this "other" Shanghai. In the concessions, a mention of "Native Shanghai" branded the speaker as somewhat barbarian, and it was definitely "bad form" to show interest in, let alone visit, that den of iniquity. It was, said one correspondent, perfectly possible for a married couple to spend an entire lifetime in "their" Shanghai without ever viewing this malodorous and contemptible neighbour.[8]

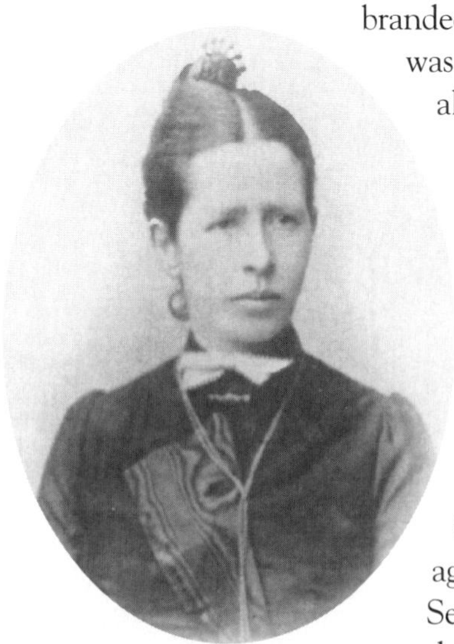

Leonora

At this point, Leonora Howard's real adventure begins. She will board another steamer, this one bound for Tientsin, some 1,600 kilometres to the north. Leaving the filthy harbour, the steamer will turn east again into the relative freshness of the Yellow Sea, heading for Tsingtao, Chefoo, and finally the Taku sandbar outside of Tientsin, where loom two long low forts. Here, at the mouth of the Pei Ho River, the steamer's captain will hire a tugboat for the perilous, winding trip inland. Although here in the north it was cooler and drier than Shanghai, the aftermath of the flood was far more in evidence. Low riverbanks led to the remains of mud villages, most of which had been swept away in the recent floods. But the industry of the northern Chinese must have filled Leonora with admiration. Survivors, temporarily housed in rude huts made of matting, old pieces of cotton or stray wooden planks, tilled every inch of available land, now that the floods had receded.

At the entrance to Tientsin, Leonora's steamboat might have stood in limbo for three days before clearance was granted. Again the harbour would be jammed, gunwale to gunwale, with every type of cargo and passenger craft imaginable. Here the stinking water was littered with the most appalling of refuse, including human feces and the occasional dead dog. The cooking smells, permeated by a strong odour of garlic and rotting fish, assaulted one's every waking moment, and the noise was unimaginable. Women banged pots and pans and yelled at the top of their lungs to merchants who poled up, offering limp brown northern cabbage salvaged from the floods.

Leonora was almost home.

Endnotes

1. Maugham, W. Somerset. *On a Chinese Screen*. Oxford: Oxford University Press, 1922, p. 83.
2. Austin, Alvyn. *Saving China: Canadian Missionaries in the Middle Kingdom, 1888-1959*. Toronto: University of Toronto Press, 1986, p. 9.
3. Miss L.A. Campbell and Miss Mary Q. Porter had been in Peking since 1872.
4. The Michigan Historical Collection, Bentley Historical Library, University of Michigan. Various Commissions and Diplomatic Missions. Box 2, China Section, No. 9. Chester Holcombe to James B. Angell, July 8, 1880.
5. Ibid.
6. Bird, Isabella. *The Yangtze Valley and Beyond*. London: Virago Press Limited, 1985, p. 24.
7. Ibid., p. 25.
8. Ibid., p. 25.

Chapter five

On the road
1877

Be strong and of a good courage;
be not afraid, neither be thou dismayed.
— Joshua 1:9

At the Taku quayside Leonora would have been met by American missionaries Reverend and Mrs. Pilcher, with whom she would reside for a few days. Because Tientsin was usually a sea of mud, owing to the vagaries of the Pei Ho River, sedan chairs were the order of the day. Constructed of light bamboo, the chairs were either open or closed, depending on locality, sex of the occupant, or social status. It is likely that in cosmopolitan Tientsin, Leonora could, even as a foreign woman, travel in an open chair without fear of molestation. A Chinese woman would be hidden behind thick silk curtains. Although the traveller's steamer trunk bumped along behind in a wheelbarrow, Leonora's precious medical bag would have rested just below the chair in a type of well made specifically for that purpose. Her back was well supported, hand-rails provided security, and her feet rested on a comfortable footboard suspended by ropes.

The chairs were attached to bamboo poles about 4 metres long that were hoisted by three coolies — two in front and one stronger man in the rear. The only difficulty was a constant shifting from one shoulder to another of a short carrying bamboo pole on which the long poles hung. This shift of weight, done simultaneously by the bearers, involved a halt to the proceedings every 90 metres or so, and gave the impression that the shoulders were suffering unbearable pain. Guilt, the Chinese knew, would certainly net a few more *cash** at the end of the journey.

*Cash was Chinese money that had a hole in it. It was carried on a string.

Leonora's procession would have been preceded by two *yamen* runners who brandished the quartet's passports, or letters of admittance to the great city, all the while shouting "In the name of the *Kuan* — In the name of the Mandarin!"* (The word *yamen* referred to a mandarin's physical offices, the place where all matters of law and commerce had final representation.) The runners, known to some as "the great unpaid," were despised by most Chinese. In large cities like Tientsin, there might be more than 1,000 of these hangers-on, earning their living both through making the aforementioned commotion on behalf of new arrivals, and through serving writs and "squeezing" the unfortunate litigants out of their last few pieces of silver. They changed at every district, after delivering up the passports or letters of introduction, and were known far and wide for their alarming habit of abandoning a traveller by selling the right (at a good profit) to bear the passports to any beggar who happened along. The Mandarin who ruled Chihli Province and Tientsin was the great Viceroy Li Hung-chang, who not only tolerated foreigners but had been known to encourage their enterprise. If a runner wanted to keep his head securely on his shoulders, he would treat these Westerners with respect.

Although the Pilchers had lived in China since 1870,[1] they had only recently moved to Tientsin from the Methodist Mission in Peking. They had to rent a home in the French concession, because the British compound, where American and Canadian missionaries normally set up housekeeping, had no vacancies. The bustling port of Tientsin was one more place for Leonora to stop, catch her breath, and have a good hot bath. She was not to know that in just two short years this rich trade centre would have a profound effect on her life.

Located about 100 kilometres east of Peking, Tientsin, as a major port, was the third most important city in China. First mentioned in the Song Dynasty writings (AD 960–1280), Tientsin rose to fame in the 14th century when grain, brought to the capital along the Grand Canal, was stored here on the way to Peking. By the 15th century Tientsin had become a garrison town with a flourishing trade and as such, became completely encircled by walls. A fort guarded the town, but nature also provided its own defence: the entire area was surrounded by malarial marshland.

In 1856, Britain had declared war on the Chinese on the pretext of an affront offered to two of its soldiers. The Chinese had fought a hopeless battle against British troops, who were reinforced by French armies. The defeated Manchu court signed treaties with Britain and France that legalized the opium trade,

*The word "mandarin" was actually Portugese, but was used by westerners to refer to all Chinese officials. The Chinese designation was kuan.

guaranteed protection to missionaries, and opened the interior to travelling "under reasonable conditions," and several new ports, including Tientsin, to foreign trade. An important stipulation was made that Christianity was to be tolerated and foreigners allowed to reside in China's great capital, Peking. By the end of the century, more concessions had been forced upon China by the Japanese, Germans, Italians, Belgians, Austro-Hungarians and Russians. During this time, commerce flourished and Tientsin developed a distinctly European flavour.

But before Leonora entered the foreign concession area, she had first to move through the gates of the "Chinese City." Tientsin was surrounded by an ancient and magnificent wall, with soaring parapets and beautifully carved gate towers with heavy doors that closed each evening at sunset. There the beauty stopped. In any season, the million residents of this thriving port sloshed through a quagmire of indescribable stench, the mud augmented every few metres by water carriers on their way to and from the great broad river or the stinking Grand Canal. Lanky yellow dogs covered in open sores skulked in alleyways just big enough for a donkey to pass through, snarling at each other over the bursting carcass of a rat that had recently made the long voyage from Singapore. Unpleasant-looking sailors made for the opium shops, and small children defecated in the streets.

Once these unsavoury elements were dealt with, the streets could actually became quite magical. Thousands of shops adorned with huge vertical signboards crowded together under strips of matting that kept the sun at bay, creating an almost twilight condition even at high noon. The signs were joyously colourful, brilliant red and gold being the hues of choice, and their fine black calligraphy announced this druggist or that tea room, this silk merchant and that seller of fine porcelain. Itinerant barbers set up their travelling shops, because even the poorest Chinese would have his forehead and eyebrows shaven, in deference to fashion decreed by his Manchu rulers. Tinkers sat cross-legged on flat stones, patiently mending well-used cooking pots. The noise was incessant.

Just as in Shanghai, Leonora Howard would suddenly find herself in fresher air, the quagmire underneath giving way to stout cobblestone streets lined with fine shade trees and imposing Western-style buildings. In stark comparison to the Chinese city, Tientsin's foreign concessions were oases. As in Shanghai, the British, French and German concession lands rolled decorously back from the river. Tientsin's Bund, though narrower than Shanghai's, was also graced with solid Victorian mansions and busy with this city's own "carriage trade."

Rather than being surrounded by high walls like the compounds Leonora would see in Peking, the huge foreign buildings in Tientsin formed their own "walls" around large courtyards. Throughout the area were dotted pretty green parks where one could sit quietly in the shade of a large maple tree — just like at home. Dominating the British Concession was China's first Western-style hotel, the fashionable Astor House, sitting on Crown Lease land negotiated by missionary John Innocent in 1863. Back then, the Astor, a far cry from its current elegance, was a type of bungalow connected to iron-roofed sheds at the back. Although initially a combination of *hong*, or company, warehouse and hotel, it had been the only place, besides a private house, that a Westerner could stay in Tientsin. It had been nicknamed the "Mud House" by those in the know. Just in front of the now-elegant entrance, Victoria Park beckoned Leonora Howard with beautifully kept lawns, shaded, winding paths, and formal flower beds in which were planted all manner of English roses. As in Shanghai, a prominent sign read "No Chinese or dogs allowed."*

Just down the street the main French compound came into view. It was one vast, continuous building, three stories high, that formed the outline of a huge square that completely surrounded a small city of its own. The buildings, beautifully finished in pink and grey stone, had many large windows, both on the outer and "courtyard" sides. Graceful columns added dignity, and huge archways on each segment of the square allowed access to both residents and tradespeople.

The Pilchers would have lived in a neat little home tucked safely within the walls of this amazing complex. Inside the compound, bright gardens boasted apple, cherry, plum and pear trees that would just be finishing their riotous burst of creamy white and rich pink bloom. And there was peace, of a sort. Apart from the sounds of the cooks banging away in the kitchens, the constant running back and forth of yelling chit-bearers, the cacophony of noise produced by carters lugging in supplies, and the continuous clip-clop of hooves — mules for the Chinese and fine ponies for the gentlemen — this place was a sea of calm for a tired traveller.

Peking beckoned, however, and Leonora would rapidly learn that in China, one first makes an offer for transportation quite casually. It will always be turned down by the provider of said transportation, who will watch the buyer walk away as if he had much more important business. The agent shouts a counter-offer, and the buyer ups his price slightly, still walking away. This process goes back and forth until the two are just within shouting distance, at which time they might begin to come to terms. These being agreed upon, it would take days before the owners of the houseboat that would take her to Peking would declare it "ready" for travel.

*Actually, a few Chinese were allowed in Victoria Park. The Viceroy Li Hung-chang, who had invested huge sums in the concession buildings, often took his family for afternoons in the park.

The houseboats that sailed up the winding Pei Ho were surprisingly comfortable. There was also a refreshing change in scenery. Where the steaming shores near Shanghai had flourished with lush sub-tropical vegetation, this country to the north was flat or slightly rolling, much like the farmland in Leonora's native Ontario. The houseboats were much larger than she, having already seen the painfully cramped quarters of the river people, had hitherto supposed. Her boat would have been about 70 metres long, with a type of hut in the middle high enough even for this tall young woman. The hut was a good enough size to house a mattress, over which foreigners placed heavy oilcloths to keep the bugs at bay, plus a small dining table and chair.

Leonora could not have made this trip alone, and under normal circumstances it would have been unheard of for a spinster to travel alone with man, missionary or not. It is therefore likely that the Pilchers accompanied her in a companion boat, filling her in on what she might find ahead. The food was edible, if not exactly palatable. But rather than face a breakfast of oily brown noodles, with lunch and dinner of the same mixed with cabbage and gristly pork, Leonora might have picnicked on the good white bread baked by the Pilchers' cook, spread thickly with bright orange persimmon jam. For lunch, canned chipped beef from the United States, warmed over a charcoal brazier, was accompanied by American biscuits with lashings of good sweet butter. The whole would be washed down with tea and condensed milk. One's meals were taken while ignoring the steady gaze of many black eyes, big and small, that peered through every chink in the cabin walls.

After three days of river travel, the two houseboats would have stopped at Tungchow for a good hot beef stew* at that town's mission station. Here the main luggage was sent on by wheelbarrow to Peking and a small sampan was rented for the last leg of the journey, back on the Grand Canal. This decision was judiciously made, for Peking's rough dusty roadways were a far cry from the clean washed pavement of Tientsin's foreign quarter.[2]

Although by 1877 it had become incredibly squalid in appearance, the Grand Canal represented China's earliest and greatest feat of engineering. The network of canals had begun far back in the Chou Dynasty (1122–1256 BC). In the year 487 BC, the state of Wu, centred around Soochow, dug the earliest canal. This connected the Huai and the Yangtze Rivers. Somewhat later, the same state constructed canals to reach the three branches of the lower Yangtze and the "five lakes." This marked the true beginning of the Grand Canal, and included an extensive irrigation system, recorded by the great historian Ssu-ma

*Beef in China was water buffalo that had grown too old to be useful in the fields.

Ch'ien, who wrote "All the canals were used for boats; and if there was sufficient water they would use it for irrigation. Peasants enjoyed the benefit ... . There were tens of thousands of ditches ... to lead the water from the canals to the fields."[3] During the Sui Dynasty (AD 589–618), China was for the first time linked politically and economically through the improvement and extension of the canal.

As it had been for thousands of years, the Grand Canal was inhabited by river folk who had seldom, if ever, set foot on land. For a middle-class girl from Eastern Ontario, even for a doctor, the life, indeed the bodily functions displayed at such close quarters, would have been alarming. The river people began each day by lighting smoky charcoal cooking fires, grass being unavailable owing to the flood, and then preparing incense sticks with solemn ritual. Boat families *kowtowed* to ancestral shrines or idols and offered bowls of *fan*, or rice, if they could afford it, before turning to their own breakfast. Women and girls with ragged, tiny bound feet did most of the work. Cooking, washing, mending and eating took up the day, until evening required more rituals in front of the shrines. If present the men, sometimes out-of-work canal coolies, sometimes opium addicts, sat in the shade, smoked, and gambled.

If this squalor was painful to a Westerner, it was more that made up for by the scenery. Intricately carved, gracefully arched bridges, and red-roofed homes with glorious curved eaves, from which hung hundreds of gaily tinkling wind chimes, might enchant the first-time visitor. Clouds of fragrant lilac, delicate mauve wisteria and bright wild roses rambled along the banks of the canal,

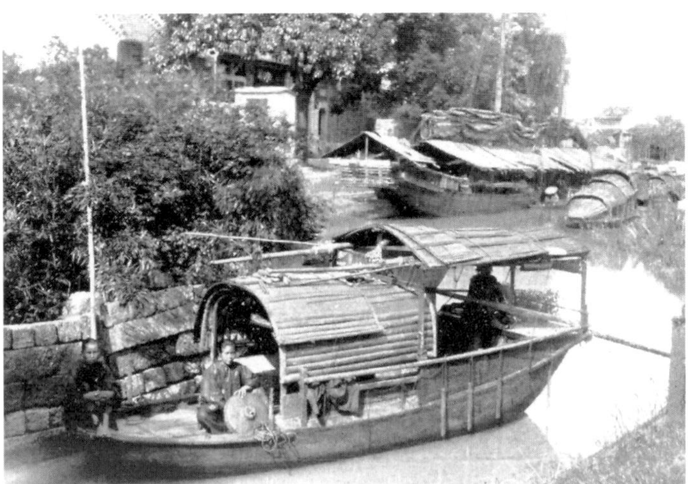

Sampan

their welcome perfume caught on tiny zephyrs of fresher air. Huge waterwheels beside the canal were worked by women, children and water buffalo. Exotic temples, farmhouses and wheat fields dotted the landscape.

But whenever boats containing foreigners stopped in the water traffic, farmers and fishermen dropped whatever they were doing and formed tight little knots of humanity that stared in flat, prolonged silence. Now for the first of what would be many thousands of times, Leonora would hear the high-pitched shriek of little children as they poked each other and yelled at the strange tall she-creature, "*Yang-kwei-tze!*," — "Foreign Devil! Foreign Devil!"

The sampans would bring the missionaries within 5 kilometres of Leonora's final destination, but that last part of the journey would be long indeed. Outside the walls of the great northern capital, she would transfer to a strange contraption known as the Peking Cart. This mule-drawn device, innocent enough to look at, was springless. Its hard wooden wheels plunged, creaking, into every pothole and bounced out again with alarming force that had thrown many unsuspecting Westerners into the ditch. In simple terms, the Peking Cart was described by more than one Westerner as the most brutal form of transport ever designed. But Leonora could not walk because women on the streets were an abomination to the male populace. She would also have been advised to stare straight ahead. This expressionless pose was quite necessary for a Westerner, particularly a woman, for any action that might show weakness to the surly mule driver, the inevitable *yamen* runners, and the beggars that grasped her cart with their filthy, clawlike hands might result in terrible disaster.

Thousands crowded this road, all headed for the magical gates, and, they hoped, the silver, of Peking. Strings of coolies, swayed along under enormous loads of raw cotton, salt, coal and foodstuffs brought in from areas that had escaped the Yellow River's wrath. Peasants pushed wheelbarrows, small children on their backs, with pitiful bundles of possessions salvaged from the flood. Little did the refugees know that they would be refused entrance to the great city.

As the sun reached its zenith Peking's glorious Ch'ien Men arches beckoned in the distance. God had delivered the doctor, almost in one piece.

Endnotes

1. *Chinese Recorder* 13, pp. 189-190.
2. The Michigan Historical Collection, Bentley Historical Library, University of Michigan. Various Commisions and Diplomatic Missions, Box 2, China Section, No. 11. The description of this route was taken from James B. Angell's correspondence to his son, August 14, 1880.
3. Chi Ch'ao-ting. *Key Economic Areas in Chinese History*. London: George Allen & Unwin Ltd., 1936, p. 66.

Chapter six

The great capital
1877

If God be with us, who can be against us?
— Romans 8:31

Peking suffered from a chronic water shortage. Most visitors were treated to stinging eyes and rasping throats. Even though it was now early summer and deep mud clung to cartwheel and boot alike, the dust remained everywhere. It filled the crevices of every house, it would settle in the folds of Leonora's clothing, and turn her red-gold hair into a grey bird's nest. For all the mud and the heat, a fierce wind still screamed down from the Gobi Desert, a wind that everyone, Chinese and foreigner alike, found a constant source of irritation. And this was not even winter, the "season of dust."*

Basically an agrarian society, China's huge population had over the centuries created a chronic drought-flood problem, particularly here in the north. A lack of knowledge about rotation planting, but particularly about reforestation, had resulted in a tragic obliteration of northern forests, and therefore a lack of wood, not only for fuel but also for economic purposes. By the 19th century, this was causing a real dilemma. Deforestation of large areas had also affected North China's climate, causing long periods of drought and with it, terrible famine. When the wood had ran out, the populace did not hesitate to grub for the roots of plants and grass for cooking fuel, and in this manner, they had denuded the soil. Thus deprived of its natural protection, the surface of the earth was exposed to dust storms that occurred several times a year, each one bearing out to the sea several million tons of fine soil. This choking, swirling grey silt still swept through Peking in early June.

---

*"The season of dust" occurred in the extremely dry winter months. During this period, the Chinese gave up attempting to keep clean and did not even bother to wash their clothes unless absolutely necessary.

Peking, with its graceful temples, enchanting gardens and mysterious mansions has for centuries so enthralled Westerners that for a moment Leonora might have forgotten the intense, smelly reality of its streets. But if there was one thing all 19th-century foreigners had in common, it was the humiliating wave of nausea that assailed them for weeks after their arrival in this wondrous city. The nausea affected men and women alike, but possibly because they were more open in their emotional outpourings, more women than men wrote that on arriving in China they had lapsed into a state of "shock and disbelief" that took months to overcome.[1] Apart from the smells, apart from the constant din, routine public beheadings — a social occasion for the Chinese — caused many a stout Western soul to faint.

In 1877, Peking was a city under siege, not from foreign invasion but from the more sinister enemies of death and disease. Not without reason was the Yellow River, *Huang Ho*, known as "China's Sorrow." Those who had survived the devastation of the flood had lost every crop. These pitiful souls were now reduced to eating grass, tree bark, even the earth itself. From the north, from the east, along the Great Wall and across barren mud flats, skeletal survivors converged with distended bellies and sunken eyes, seeking life in the very garbage outside Peking's walls. Mothers who had crooned to their offspring last month now slapped sons into the art of begging and kept a sharp eye out for men who would buy their worthless daughters. Men sold wives and concubines into slavery. New baby girls were strangled or drowned in the night.

But not all of Peking's beggars were refugee peasants. The professionals, ragged, filthy, riddled with lice and fleas, were ruled by ferocious beggar kings who sent them to work the shops — and the missionaries — for protection money. Most merchants were glad to pay some small amount, because respectable customers would refuse to enter the premises with such vermin whining for *cash*. Old China Hands, when challenged by the rogues, would most likely refuse to pay, preferring confrontation over compensation.

But if the doctor had dared to look up for a moment, her breath would be taken away, for just up the road was the gorgeously hued Temple of Heaven. This masterpiece of engineering had neither nail nor bolt — each beautifully carved piece of wood fitting into another with awesome precision. Tier after tier of gracefully curving roof soared to the sky and hundreds of the faithful burned pieces of incense or paper money in honour of their ancestors.

Peking, a "closed city," was less used to foreigners than cosmopolitan Shanghai. Leonora would be stared at mercilessly and even pinched, poked, and prodded whenever her little cortège came to a stop. Travelling in an open cart on the streets of Peking often entailed this type of harassment, but an adventurous spirit could not fail to be caught up in the vivid life of these surprisingly spacious boulevards. The well-fed residents of the capital* spilled in happy waves onto the streets, so that in some places the broad thoroughfares narrowed considerably, but here, unlike Tientsin, there was ample room for the carts, rickshaws and sedan chairs to manoeuvre. But like Tientsin, like Shanghai, Leonora could glimpse to the right, then the left, those darker, narrower streets that were more like tunnels, with poles laid from roof to roof, covered with straw mats to keep the sun at bay. In these alleyways the geomancers shook long tall sticks in wooden cups, telling fortunes and consulting the stars, opium dens beckoned the rich, the poor, but always the weak, and age-old chemists' shops proffered ginseng, tigers' bones, and bears' gallbladders for use as aphrodisiacs.

Now the missionaries and the mules began to move through market streets that rang as much with laughter as shouts of outrage, as servants of the rich, middle-class husbands and honourable eldest sons bartered for imported southern food. Although some diplomats insisted that Peking's selection of vegetables and fruit was poor,[2] Leonora would pass hundreds of stalls laden with strange and delectable produce. Tender bamboo shoots, smooth shining eggplant, heavy orange yams and rich red radishes sat beside baskets of gleaming rice that had replaced the flooded northern wheat. Bean sprouts, almonds, succulent smoked duck were haggled over, sometimes for an hour or more. The young doctor would also be treated to a chorus of squawking chickens, protesting pigs, and the unique wails and clangs of each street vendor loudly proclaiming the excellence of his product.

When the shoppers tired, they stopped at any of the hundreds of tea shops that lined the streets of Peking. Here, amid raucous games of *mah-johng*, they would savour small squares of sweet browned bean curd or suck noisily at the firm pink prawns carried in from the seaside near Tientsin. Prawn shells and chicken bones were tossed on the greasy floors and happy belches resounded. Everywhere on the streets vendors sold piping hot vegetable patties of beans, chopped cucumbers, or sweet potato and wheat cakes containing savoury fried onion.

*As Peking was a closed city and home to many aristocrats, as well as the royal family, the residents generally had enough money to buy food that was imported from areas that had not been stricken by drought.

Outside the city walls, the famine victims begged for *kuh-li*, or coolie work in the city for a few cash or for one bowl of thin gruel per day. Many simply perished at the gates. The name *kuh-li*, or "bitter strength," had come about because the bearers eventually developed a constant grimace from the loads they carried, and their teeth became bared in a bitter parody of a smile. This year, hundreds of flood refugees had turned to coolie work for fan, or rice, although the amateurs' raw red sores and hot white blisters gave them away as strangers. Although lowest on the social ladder, coolies had never been slaves and carried no "untouchable" stigma as did their brothers in India.

Floods along the Yellow River were frequent, but this year's disaster had caused unusual destruction. Weak attempts to curb the course of China's rivers had availed nothing. This was due to a lack of engineering skill and the dishonesty of the mandarins who supervised the work. While the ancient Chinese had been world pioneers in irrigation, there was an urgent need to deepen and broaden China's countless artificial waterways, employing modern engineering methods to remove rapids and other obstructions to navigation, and to construct reservoirs to control flood waters.[3] It is significant that since 1644 the originally adventurous Manchus, by assimilating almost completely into the Han Chinese way of life, had cracked down on innovation to the extent that intelligent men did little but study Confucius,

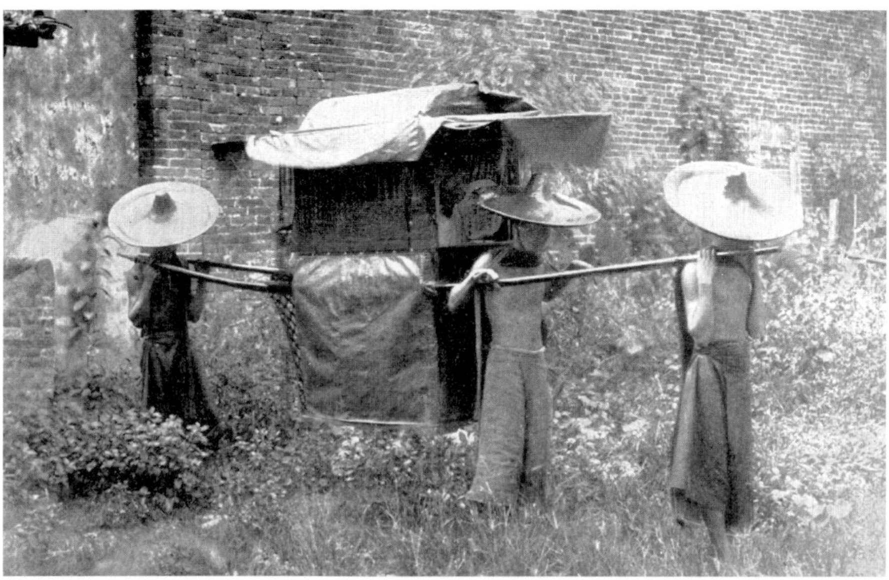

Sedan chair

write poetry, practise calligraphy, and keep their mouths shut. The Mandarins, almost all Manchu, suffered from political myopia to the extent that armies, traditional bastions of engineering, were effete and disorganized. In fact, the profession of soldier was by now held in such contempt that indeed no man of ability would lower himself to take up such a career. The Empress Dowager's Bannermen, who "ran" China's armies, were prohibited from taking up real professions, and as such were indolent, arrogant and, worst of all, ignorant.[4]

But back to Leonora's first sights of Peking. The street widened and the crowds thinned. Just short of her destination, she probably had a tantalizing glimpse of the red-tiled rooftops of the "Forbidden City" where the Emperor and his Dowager guardian reigned in isolated splendour. A mile down the road a large building with a prominent cross proclaimed that Christ had entered China.

Endnotes

1. Hunter, Jane. *The Gospel of Gentility - American Women Missionaries in Turn-of-the-Century China*. New Haven: Yale University Press, 1984, pp. 1-2.
2. The Michigan Historical Collection, Bentley Historical Library, University of Michigan. Various Commissions and Diplomatic Missions. Box 2, China Section, No. 9. Chester Holcombe to James B. Angell, July 8, 1880.
3. Smith, Arthur H. *The Uplift of China*. New York: Forward Mission Study Courses. Young People's Missionary Movement of the United States and Canada, 1907, pp. 17-18.
4. Warner, Marina. *The Dragon Empress: Life and Times of Tz'u-hsi, 1835-1908, Empress Dowager of China*. London: Cardinal, 1974, p. 21.

Chapter seven

Scattering the seed
1877–1879

If people who are like mud and wood are useless and stupid, how much more the real mud and wood?
— Ting Chin Si, Deaconess, Ku Cheng, 1877

The Methodist mission that Leonora would call home was attractive, spacious and comfortable. Its political importance was represented by the chapels that opened onto the street. Each chapel prominently displayed the Chinese Emperor's proclamation concerning foreign treaty rights. The compound, situated in the Tartar, or Manchu-occupied city, consisted of two pieces of property, on the oldest of which was built "two moderately fair, one-story brick residences ... ," a girls' boarding school, and a residence belonging to the WFMS. For white people only, there was the domestic chapel, "a very pleasant, good-sized building, used for the more private and orderly services of the Church members." On the second piece of property, "unfortunately separated from the first by two or three intervening Chinese properties," there was first, a very comfortable and well-built brick residence, and second, a neat and pleasant home and comfortable hospital and dispensary.[1] Leonora would share the residence with Dr. Lucinda Coombs, Miss L.A. Campbell, and Mary Q. Porter.

The mission had opened early in 1869, when Reverends L.N. Wheeler and H.H. Lowrie and their families were transferred from Foochow. The following year they secured premises in the southeast corner of the Tartar City, near one of the city gates. Toward the close of 1870, the mission was reinforced by the addition of Reverends G.R. Davis and L.W. Pilcher. In 1871, Maria Browne and Mary Q. Porter were appointed by the WFMS to work with Chinese women and girls. Their arrival was, however, delayed until spring of 1872. In December 1875, Miss L.A. Campbell arrived and plunged into the study of the Chinese language. She would later befriend and translate for Leonora. In 1871, after meeting with much hostility from officials and the anti-foreign segment of the population, a preaching chapel was exchanged[2] for a much larger one "on another principal street to the West, on which a new chapel has been built for preaching to the heathen and on which there is ample accommodation for boys' and girls' schools." One year later the street chapel previously belonging to the Presbyterians was procured. In that same year, Reverend G.R. Davis opened a branch of the mission in Tientsin. Lucinda Coombs commenced medical work in 1873, and a hospital for women and children was opened in autumn 1875. The staff of ladies connected with the WFMS was further increased when Clara Cushman arrived in 1878.[3]

Lucinda Coombs was a pious soul, an American orphan who had supported and educated herself from an early age. According to one biographer, Lucinda had consecrated her life to God, and the language of her heart was "my Father, be thou the guide of my youth," as, when her father and mother forsook her, the Lord had presumably taken her up. After a religious conversion sometime in her teens, Lucinda had one goal — to enter missionary work in India. As we already know, the WFMS sent her to China instead.

Like Leonora, Lucinda had taught school before entering medical school. After receiving "the call" she attended the Cazenovia Seminary in the United States, where she stayed consistently at the head of her classes, graduating with the highest honours. With no family to take up her time, she had plunged into the religious life with great fervour, toiling relentlessly while other students went on vacation. She was determined to live up to her motto of "Excelsior."

On hearing about the value of a medical education for female missionaries, Lucinda had decided to secure such education herself, "leaving nothing undone which would aid in qualifying her to the utmost for usefulness in her future work." Thus it was that on graduation from the seminary, she entered a women's medical college in Philadelphia, with the intense interest and most probably the financial support of the WFMS. Lucinda Coombs had sailed for Peking on June 5, 1873, and was the first woman physician to set foot in China.[4]

Like other missionaries before them, Lucinda, Maria Brown and Mary Q. Porter found that the growth of "the work" had not been rapid, but like others in the field who depended on funding from home, each reported exceedingly encouraging results. The Misses Brown and Porter had opened a girls' school soon after arriving in China. This institution had continued with varying numbers and success, and inevitably, not a little good seed scattered among "the heathen." When Leonora arrived that warm summer's day, the North China Mission school boasted 17 Chinese students, three of whom had become members of the Methodist church. Several other children, reported the missionaries, were "earnestly seeking to do the will of the Master."

Not to pass up any good opportunity, the Americans ensured that meetings for Chinese women, particularly those whose children attended the school, were held weekly. Although the Chinese women had never heard of Christianity, several had apparently given good evidence of conversion. One, wrote Mary Porter, had actually come several hundred kilometres to learn the doctrines, so that she could "be prepared to tell the wonderful story of the cross to her idolatrous neighbors."

The women, however, came as much for socializing as for proselytizing, and once they were ensconced in these congenial, female-run premises, it was often difficult to get them to leave. To the vast amusement of Dr. Coombs, Miss Porter and Miss Campbell, who had run the gauntlet before, these lovely, curious Chinese women would immediately crowd around newcomers like Leonora, plucking at her Western garments, feeling her wiry red-gold hair, touching the lids of her huge round eyes, and finally lifting her long skirts to see if she had two legs, just like Chinese women.

With all these intriguing sights, plus the novel experience of leaving the isolation and strictures of a Chinese home, it was little wonder that conversation took precedence over conversion. So the children, being far more impressionable, were better to focus on in order to advance Christ's cause. By 1877, a Peking auxiliary to the WFMS had been formed, in which the "mites," or children of missionaries, the offspring of Chinese Christian women, and some of the little orphaned schoolgirls were given the job of sending the Gospel to those who had not yet received it, a technique used again, almost 100 years later, during the Communist Party's Cultural Revolution.

Doctors Lucinda Coombs and Leonora Howard would set major precedents during their years in China. Their medical work was, far more than Bible classes, an efficient agent for reaching and teaching Chinese women about the freedom and dignity allowed by Christianity. Although Leonora would be more secular in her approach, Lucinda, throughout her professional labours, "never failed to point her patients to the Great Physician." What did it matter that when one intelligent Chinese was asked if she understood the Gospel, she replied "Oh yes! Our gods are made of clay and yours are made of wood!" Dr. Coombs was truly earnest in her desire to help downtrodden Chinese women.

While Leonora was still settling in, Mary Porter was sent home for treatment of her eyes. Happily for everyone, this practical, Chinese-speaking missionary returned to Peking in midsummer 1878. For in that same period, Dr. Coombs married Reverend Andrew Strittmater, whom she had met on the way to China in 1873. It had been exactly five years — the mandatory years of spinsterhood — that Lucinda had been in the service of the WFMS, and like many other WFMS members, she leapt at the chance for the freedom of a home and family.

Andrew Strittmater was from Pennsylvania, and had been brought up by genuinely religious parents in the Methodist Episcopal Church. The reverend had, in fact, been something of a child prodigy when it came to decent, God-fearing behaviour. His habits in youth were "of the steadiest and purest kind" and "Wanton, cruel, or sinful sports, such as please most boys, had no charms whatever for him ... " Like Lucinda, Andrew truly believed, and when asked at the age of 19 whether he had read the Bible throughout, he reportedly smiled, "though weeping," and said that he had read it 10 times. Lucy and Andrew were indeed kindred spirits, for as a missionary, "he was every thing that could be desired ... strong in body, clear in mind, and pure in heart."

Sadly, this deeply religious marriage ended in tragedy. With Leonora now on board, Lucinda and her husband moved far away to Kiu Kiang to further serve their Lord. Poor Andrew was "industrious — too industrious," and through overwork in his college days, and by overwork and exposure in open boats and in an unfriendly country, the seeds of his death were quickly sown. When urged to return home to save himself, Andrew said "I think we ought to show the heathen that we can die for them as well as live for them." Finally he consented to return to America when he felt useless in the missionary field. The lonely orphan Lucinda Coombs Strittmatter accompanied her husband back to Ohio. Andrew died in 1880 and his wife did not return to China.

After Lucinda left, life at the mission went on, and apart from overwork in the "hospital," Leonora's own existence was fairly comfortable. We do know that she ate very well indeed. Food was one indulgence that everyone allowed themselves, being, as it were, stuck on the other side of the world. Beef and mutton were usually available to the foreigners, the latter being sold in Muslim shops that had served Peking for centuries.

In a closed community it is well to follow custom, and Leonora would learn that most Westerners refused food prepared in the Chinese fashion, unless compelled to eat it on the road. Later on, when Canadian missionaries arrived at the China Inland Mission, they wrote that "The fare is good and sufficient. For breakfast we get good bread ... toast, porridge, or some meal, tea with condensed milk, meat or fish." For dinner, there was meat or fowl, vegetables, potatoes, pudding, oranges and nuts. At teatime, the missionaries ate fish or meat, "sometimes an egg or two," with bread, butter and treacle.[5] At times it seemed as if everyone was trying to outdo each other when entertaining: roast chicken and the famed Shuenwei ham, mutton, green peas and red currant jelly was the fare offered to a traveller in one missionary station. This particular meal was rounded out with thin pancakes and Yunnan cheese, the whole being washed down with claret, champagne, port and cordial Medoc.[6] It was a wonder that no one became fat.

Leonora Howard's 27th birthday, her first away from home, was darkened by the death of a new and close friend. In early May 1878, Miss Campbell was prostrated by malignant fever, and after a brief illness "was not." Leonora was devastated. By the slim blue light of her kerosene lamp, she wrote that "The last three months have brought sad days to the North China Mission. Death has invaded our ranks and borne away one who seemed indispensable to our work here. Miss Campbell was a great deal to me." Together, the two young women had held "hospital services," and when Leonora was called to visit outpatients, Miss Campbell had accompanied her as interpreter. Her friend, wrote Leonora, had been tremendously successful in communicating with the Chinese, as "Invariably, the people received us cordially, listened respectfully, and sometimes eagerly, while she presented to them the one true God." This first of many colleagues' deaths must have been a terrible blow for the young Canadian.

To the women of the WFMS in America, the loss of Miss Campbell meant far more than an emotional cry in the wilderness. Each missionary in the field was in fact a serious financial investment. After she had been "numbered among the glorified — the blood-washed of all nations!," the late Miss Campbell presented a problem, for first her body would have to be shipped

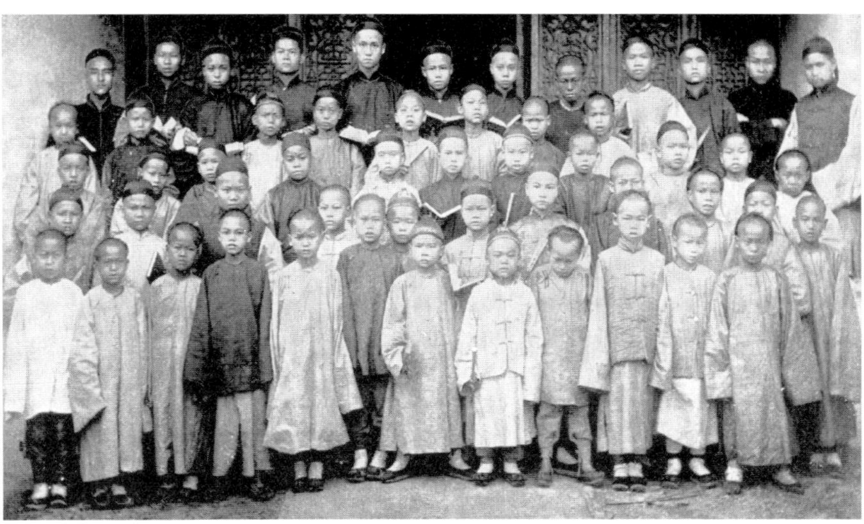

Typical mission pupils

home, at not inconsiderable expense, and second, she would have to be replaced, and quickly. "Dark, indeed, this shadow for our mission in Peking!" wrote the recording secretary. "So intimately connected with the work, and so essential for its successful prosecution, in the estimation of those most deeply interested in its greatest prosperity, that her sudden removal was wellnigh overwhelming to her colaborers [sic]." Whether or not it was overwhelming to Leonora was a moot point: Miss Campbell had been fluent in Chinese, and it would take another five or so years before anyone could hope to replace her.

With both Lucinda Coombs and Miss Campbell gone, Leonora now ran the hospital alone while Mary Porter ran the school. Luckily for all concerned, Miss Campbell's place was quickly taken up by the ebullient Clara Cushman, who retained "all the glow of enthusiasm which inspired her when she first gave herself to this work." Clara had, Leonora wrote, expressed the deepest gratitude that she had been permitted to occupy "such a pleasant place in the world-wide vineyard of the Master." Maybe she had arrived in early autumn — the most beautiful time of year in Peking.

Clara, of course, spoke not a word of Chinese, and Mary Porter, after only six years on the job, was now the only remaining Old China Hand in the mission. Mary and Clara would remain in China for many years, for they were extremely dedicated souls, not to mention astute businesswomen. Even in her earliest reports to the WFMS, Mary was full of glowing accounts of Chinese women converting their sisters one and all, though this was hardly the case. But her tactics for fundraising worked remarkably well: while on furlough in America, she had impressed the WFMS members immensely by singing *When he cometh, to make up his jewels* — in Chinese. After this, wrote one correspondent, "touching allusion was made (about) the great sacrifice and sorrow of a mother in giving a daughter to go to foreign lands." The audience sang, "with overflowing eyes,"

"Were the whole realm of nature mine
That were a present far too small;
Love so amazing, so divine,
Demands my soul, my life, my all."

In the end, it was people like Mary Porter and Clara Cushman who kept the real missionary enterprise running smoothly. In order to keep the flow of much-needed dollars steady, they often sent back translations of letters from "Christian helpers" by which they meant Chinese converts. One such letter, from the Ku Cheng deaconess Ting Chin Si, read, in part:

> This Quarter I have gone to my relatives' and friends' houses to sell books and to teach. I find that the people know to distinguish between good

and evil. One day I was passing ... a *greatly-believing-idols* man's house. A woman inside called me in and said, "Give you to see. Can the idols hear and answer?" I replied, "Have you not heard persons rebuking the lazy use the words, "You are made of mud and wood? If people who are *like* mud and wood are exceedingly useless and stupid, how much more the *real* mud and wood useless! Can that (idol) hear and answer?

The woman in question apparently became very angry and ordered the deaconess from her home, but soon thereafter, her child sickened and died, and the woman's husband took an axe and cut the idol in pieces. Unfortunately, several other families had a share in this idol, and they insisted that the destroyer provide a new one. Although he did so, Deaconess Ting reported that the man and his wife now "hear me teach the doctrines and desire to put away all bad customs."

With this kind of emotional report emanating from the field, Mary Porter and her colleagues had done quite well in the last few years. By 1877, the WFMS owned the following Peking real estate:

Home and School	\$4,487.17
Hospital and Dispensary	\$5,621.82[7]

From 17 students the year previous, the North China Mission School became in 1878 increasingly prosperous, numbering at the close of the year some 30 girls. For the last half of that year, the missionaries decided that there were so many new students that the school building was far too small to accommodate them all. Thus began what remained for many missionaries an almost constant pastime of building and renovation. The Peking missionaries decided to enlarge the school building before the rainy season commenced. In order to have the work of demolishing and building going on without interrupting studies, the women quite reasonably moved the school into the late Miss Campbell's rooms. But, said Mary Porter, so steadily had the numbers continued to increase that the school had, by the end of the year, already outgrown the house as enlarged, and further funds would be needed for larger accommodations. As expected, the money came from somewhere across the ocean and teachers, students and Bible women alike delighted in a new, well-lit schoolroom with real wooden floors.

Mary Porter, still determined that mothers as well as children should receive the benefit of The Word, began to devote one to two hours a day to instructing six Chinese women, all of whom, reported Leonora, had been under instruction for several years and all of whom read "quite well." This was highly unusual and a great breakthrough, for the vast majority of Chinese women were totally illiterate. One of these women was a young widow, a Christian, who assisted Leonora in the dispensary and the hospital wards. She was the first Chinese "nurse" to work on behalf of her sisters, but her name was not recorded.

"The work" itself was arduous, for news of the woman doctor spread like wildfire. Hundreds lined the courtyards each day in the hope that the Foreign Devil physician could cure their ailments, set their broken bones, and bring sight to those who could not see. The hospital zone bore strange contrast to the noisome outer city, because the "wards" — dim, dirt-floored shacks — were almost silent. The Chinese, with a patience borne of thousands of years, waited for hours and sometimes for days before Leonora could see them. They came on foot, by wheelbarrow, by richly embroidered closed sedan chair, and they waited. They played *mah-jong*, they brewed tea, they bounced their babies on their laps, and they waited. Sometimes entire families set up camp in the courtyards, cooking their meals and refusing to leave the patient, just in case the Foreign Devil medicine would be used to make gold out of the loved one's liver! But still they came, and Leonora's days became hard and long.

Although Leonora worked in Peking, she also spent a great deal of time on the road, or more appropriately, the beaten track. Itinerant missionary doctors and dentists set up shop at any convenient (non-hostile) stop, such as under a tree or near the steps of a temple. One character, called the "Black-Bearded Barbarian of Formosa,"* fancied himself a doctor, and would "take (a) stand in an open space ... and, after singing a hymn or two, proceed to extract teeth and then preach the message of the Gospel."[8]

Leonora's North China Mission included four circuits. Tsunhuachow, 160 kilometres to the east was "the only Christian agency in all the vast eastern region stretching away to the (Chihli) gulf"; Tsangchow was 160 kilometres south of Tientsin; Nankung some 322 kilometres southwest of Tientsin, and Taian, still farther south, was "the only Methodist work in Shantung Province." Leonora, accompanied by at least one other missionary, made field trips either by the hated Peking cart or on the recalcitrant back of an equally hated mule. Now and again she was even "backpacked" by wiry coolies who blithely hefted the young doctor with little more than a quiet grunt. During these trips the women spent many an uncomfortable night in country inns that were little more than filthy hovels teeming with lice and bedbugs.

Chinese inns were common in Chihli Province, as there was an enormous itinerant population. Touts stood in each doorway, crying the merits of their premises in voices that some missionaries felt would shatter glass, were there any glass around. At each inn, the hired coolies conducted lengthy conversations with each tout, as often as not moving on, saying "inn no good for *tai-tais*. Very bad joss," by which they meant that their "squeeze" from the innkeeper

*The Rev. George Leslie McKay.

was not large enough. By nightfall, when travelling anywhere was dangerous, Leonora might enter a courtyard that looked more promising than most. The floor, though quite clean, was naked earth, but, she would note gratefully, it had packed quite dry in the arid northern air. At a counter inside the entrance, piles of Chinese bedding were stacked ready for hire. Leonora and all other foreign travellers carried oil-cloth sheets to cover these "mattresses," which literally swarmed with bedbugs, and most probably she set up her own campbed, rather than sleep on those foul cotton pads.

In the courtyards, other travellers who had been smoking, drinking tea and noisily gambling at rough outdoor tables often would fall into the now-familiar silence at her appearance. One by one the men would rise and slowly walk in her direction. Soon a tightly knit crowd would gather around Leonora and her companions, then all of a sudden shouting and gesticulation would break with the shattering force of a summer storm. Dirty hands formed fists that shook menacingly in the dusk and high-pitched screams of "Child Eaters! Foreign Devils!" filled the courtyard. The missionaries' hired coolies and the innkeeper would have to shove their way through the crowd, yelling as loudly as anyone, and quickly propel the women into a small dank room, the only light being provided by a limp wick set in a saucer of rank-smelling oil. Slamming the door against the mob, Leonora would shove one of the rude, straw-covered bedsteads under the latch. This fairly common experience had made more than one woman sick with fear, but on the whole it was all talk and no action, and very few were actually killed.

When Leonora and her colleagues approached a village, their runners marched importantly ahead waving the necessary "passports" signed by Li Hung-chang, the legendary Viceroy of Chihli Province. But now the doctor would face another problem. Inside the walls, under a tree, wherever the missionaries set up shop, the Chinese women, like those at the Peking mission, would grab at their hair, finger their clothing and touch their faces, all the while chattering excitedly as they tried yet again to look up the long American skirts. All this said, the missionary women were often luckier than their male colleagues. For one thing they were molested far less often. For another, they were allowed to build schools and hold clinics where many men were forbidden to tread or were even murdered for their efforts. After all, noted one District prefect, they were only women and as such, they were not worth the bother.

Some of the most appalling problems arose from the Chinese custom of binding little girls' feet, to create three-inch "golden lilies" that apparently were of great sexual interest to men. Adventurer Isabella Bird quoted Dr. Wells Williams as saying "the practice ... is more an inconvenient than a dangerous custom," but, said Miss Bird, "I have never seen a hospital in China without some case ... of extreme danger to the foot or great toe, but of ulcers or gangrene, involving absolute loss by amputation."

There was no specific age for binding feet, but upper-class children usually had it done before they were five years old. The poorer classes waited until betrothal or between the ages of seven and nine. Foot-binding was much more painful as the little girls became older, and the treatment of the big toe was different. Young girls had four toes doubled under the foot, with the big toe laid on top. Older girls suffered much more agony. Toes would be violently bent under the foot and bandaged in that position, to the extent that often tendons were ruptured.

Women in China had to bind their feet each day, or the "beauty" of the shape would be lost. The whole process of deforming them was carried out by carefully regulated bandaging. As a result, the muscles of a girl's calf would atrophy, and from knee to foot there would be folds of superfluous skin.

In between endless days of amputating little legs, dispensing morphine, lancing boils, and removing cataracts — a common problem in China — in between writing reports to the WFMS, and in between budgeting for supplies and living expenses, Leonora pored over the mandatory "Course of Study for Missionaries," which included intensive study of the Mandarin language. For her first year on the job, she would cover:

The Gospel of John
Wade's Forty Exercises and Ten Dialogues (Chinese)
Write radicals and characters in Forty Exercises
Translate ten sentences from Chinese into English
Translate ten sentences from English into Chinese
Converse with (the) teacher, (and)
Write short address to heathen."

Her second year entailed a study of:

Matthew, Mark and Luke
Wade's Hundred Lessons
Pilgrim's Progress (two volumes)
T'ien Tao Shuo Yuan (Mandarin)
writing characters in Matthew and Hundred Lessons and
writing sermon to Christians.

Language study was imperative for all missionaries, including wives. But limited expectations for the latter, combined with their own self-doubts, often led them to restrict their studies. In early days, particularly before the birth of a child, a couple would receive equal tuition and lead quite egalitarian lives. Later in the 19th century, however, the mission boards set less stringent examinations for wives. One pregnant young wife wrote that the head of the school was "very tender" with her, ruling some with an iron hand, but never berating her. The impossibility of her learning Chinese to any great extent was obvious in the fact that she was not allowed to read or write: all she could do was talk.

Leonora plunged into language training as soon as she arrived in Peking. The training took the most part of a year and although others were expected to be proficient before they ventured into the field, she, as a physician, had to fit language lessons in between patients. Because learning the tonal variations and complexities of the language was quite exhausting, training was split up during the day. One Canadian recruit would write:

> We all meet together, sing a hymn, read a chapter, expositions by Mr. Baller ... exhortations, prayer and a hymn. After this, prayers in Chinese in the chapel, at which eight or more (Chinese) are present; 9.0–10.30 private study of Chinese, 10.30–11.30. Chinese class with Mr. Baller, 12.30 dinner. Time between class and dinner for study, and prayer. Prayer for the provinces immediately after dinner till about 1.50. ... a Chinese teacher from 2 till 3 or 3.30, and private study at Chinese till 5.0.

The missionaries, besides opportunistic merchants in the treaty ports, were almost the only foreigners to even attempt Chinese. Diplomats, if they spoke to Chinese people at all, used the bastardized "pidgin," e.g., the "lookee smart get missy" type of thing. Some Westerners who could not learn Chinese convinced themselves that this was the only English the Chinese themselves were capable of learning. Many Chinese, who understood English perfectly, laughed behind their sleeves and went along with the Westerners' arrogance. This pretence of ignorance was particularly helpful for many household staff, many of whom, as a matter of course, robbed their employers blind.

Owing to the hundreds of dialects spoken throughout China, communicating with women in the field was another obstacle. Leonora solved this by enlisting and educating Chinese "Bible Women" who spoke one of the major languages, such as the Peking dialect, as well as one or more village dialects. Although educational and medical work was, by some, regarded as the mainstay of China mission work, world evangelism remained the ultimate goal of those raising the funds at home. Even though she picked up the Peking dialect quite quickly, Leonora depended on local interpreters to spread The Word on the road.

The lessons would go on for eight years, becoming more complex with each year of Chinese study. This was, of course, assuming that Leonora would not, like Dr. Lucy Coombs, get married at the first chime of that five-year gong of freedom, and give up her WFMS work to be, simply, a missionary wife.

So far, Leonora's contacts with the Chinese had been limited to treating poor and indigent women and children. She had seen the filth, gagged at the smell of open sewers, tended lepers and had mud slung at her by toothless vagabonds. But back in the Tartar City, behind immense red doors, there lived another China. Behind those huge studded doors lived the infant Emperor Kuang-hsu and his guardian, the 53 year-old Empress Dowager, Tz'u-hsi.

Endnotes

1. Barclay, Wade Crawford. *History of Methodist Missions*. Part Two, Volume Three. New York: Board of Missions and Church Extension of the Methodist Church, 1949, p. 414.
2. In this portion of the *Chinese Recorder*, someone has inserted "... exchanged in 1880", but then switches back to 1871. The author can only assume this is a mistake on the writer's part.
3. *Chinese Recorder* 15, p. 309.
4. Woman's Foreign Missionary Society of the Methodist Episcopal Church. Executive Committee, Fifth Meeting, 1881, pp. 34-39.
5. Austin, Alvyn J. *Saving China: Canadian Missionaries in the Middle Kingdom, 1888-1959*. Toronto: University of Toronto Press, 1986, p. 13.
6. Morrison, G.E. (Chinese). *An Australian in China*. Sydney, Australia: Angus and Robertson (Publishers) Pty. Ltd., 1972, p. 147.
7. *Minutes* of the Eighth Annual Meeting of the General Executive Committee of the Woman's Foreign Missionary Society of the Methodist Episcoal Church. Minneapolis, Minnesota: Centenary M.E. Church, May 1877, p. 14.
8. Austin, *Saving China*, p. 33.

Chapter eight

Empress
1877

Although I have heard much about Queen Victoria ...
I don't think her life is half as interesting ... as mine!
— Tz'u-hsi, Empress Dowager of China

Tz'u-hsi, the Motherly, Auspicious, Orthodox, Heaven-blessed, Prosperous, All-nourishing, Brightly-manifest, Calm, Sedate, Perfect, Long-lived, Respectful, Reverend, Worshipful, Illustrious and Exalted, lived in a pink-walled pavilion in the Forbidden City. Her daily walks were taken in peaceful courtyards filled, as the seasons progressed, with soft clouds of cherry, peach and plum blossoms, graceful mauve wisteria, heavy gold acacia and, when autumn's nip arrived, a profusion of scarlet, magenta and bright orange chrysanthemums. At night, huge brass cauldrons and bright paper lanterns lit up graceful soaring bridges and intricately carved marble steps, and reflected the shimmering robes of 3,000 eunuchs and another 3,000 women — concubines, other court ladies, serving women and various hangers-on. After nightfall, all guards, princes and other court advisers had to leave the grounds. In the hours of love, the Emperor could be the only sexually intact man in the entire palace.

The Empress Dowager's apartments were simply but sumptuously furnished with red silk-cushioned benches, heavy rosewood chairs and low shining black tables. An intricately carved blackwood *k'ang*, or bed, was laid with a thick felt pad and three soft mattresses covered with imperial yellow brocade. Her pillows were filled with rose petals or fragrant tea leaves. The bed curtains, even her sheets, were of the softest yellow silk, and a spread of rich yellow satin was embroidered with soaring gold dragons and soft blue clouds. A portrait of Queen Victoria stood by her bed.

Tz'u-hsi normally rose between midnight and 3 am. After a bowl of hot milk sweetened with honey and almonds, and usually some lotus-root porridge, she would be bathed and dressed by her ladies-in-waiting. If an audience were to be held (Westerners were appalled at having to appear just before dawn), she wore a yellow satin gown embroidered with pink peonies and an elaborate headdress with pearl and jade flowers on each side, with a precious jade phoenix in the centre. This costume was as much for her own pleasure as for show to her staff, because all audiences were conducted from behind a yellow silk curtain, through which Tz'u-hsi could see, yet not be seen.

As a widow, Tz'u-hsi could not wear makeup, which might, in fact, have accounted for her longevity in those days of disease and early death. Like their 16th-century sisters in the French court, upper-class Chinese women often poisoned their systems by applying white lead to their faces. The Empress Dowager, knowing that her dark Manchu complexion was not attractive in China, sprayed her face with a mixture of glycerine and honeysuckle, then dusted a bit of pinkish rice powder on and rouged her bottom lip and cheeks to disguise the light makeup. Her breath was "sweetened" with betel nuts that stained what was left of her teeth dark red.

Tz'u-hsi loved clothes. Her sumptuous Dragon Robe, embroidered with seed pearls and intricately carved coral, was imperial yellow with red, blue and her favourite purple stripes at the hem. Her audience cape, which became famous, was covered with 3,500 large gleaming pearls. Pearl and jade bracelets graced her wrists, and heavy jade rings adorned her hands. Her ring and little fingernails were covered with intricately carved gold and jade nail protectors. For centuries, mandarins had shown their wealth by growing their nails to ridiculous lengths, simply to show the rest of the world that they did no labour for themselves. For practicality's sake, however, the thumb and first two fingers were trimmed to usable length. The mother of the Middle Kingdom, who was an accomplished artist and calligrapher, would find it difficult to hold a brush otherwise.

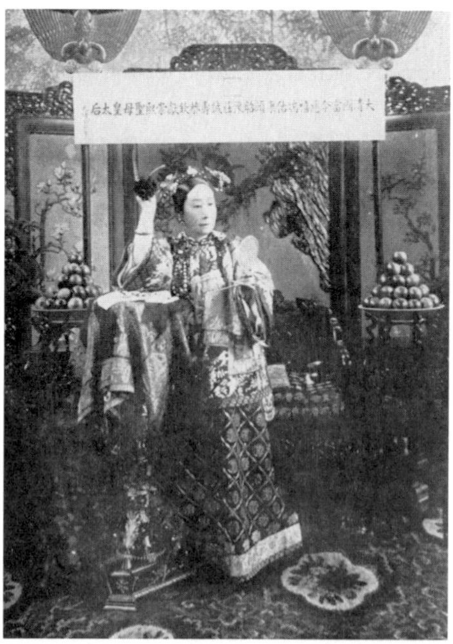

Empress Dowager Tz'u-hsi

The Middle Kingdom was, of course, called China by Westerners.

The name had been derived from the ancient house of Tsin, or Ch'in, a powerful family in Northwest China. The Chow dynasty under which Confucius flourished (551–478 BC) lasted from 1050 to 247 BC. In this period, and the subsequent period of "warring states," the great house of Ch'in was dreaded by the rest of the Middle Kingdom. In 221 BC, the prince of this house, Shih Hwang, proclaimed himself Emperor and made the vast territories into one empire. Tragically, this despot destroyed the ancient books to blot out remembrance of former sovereigns. He was also responsible for beginning the Great Wall to keep out the Tartar tribes of the North. China was also known as Sin, Chin, Sinae, and Sinim.

In addition, the Chinese were known as Seres, or "silk men," hence *Serica* or silk garments became the Latin term for silk. In the Middle Ages, China was known as *Cathay*, a name derived from the Ki-Tans, or Khi-Tai, another tribe that ruled in China. It will be remembered that Columbus originally set out for Cathay and *Zipangu*, or Japan, when he bumped into what is now America. The Chinese themselves retained the name of *Han*, the dynasty that succeeded the Ch'in, or of *Tang*, a dynasty that ruled in 620 AD.

The Manchus had swept to power in 1644 and today, in 1877, they still ruled this vast and turbulent empire. Tz'u-hsi, Empress Dowager, was naturally a member of the Manchu ruling class. She had been born Lan Kuei (Little Orchid) in 1835, on the tenth day of the tenth moon. Her father, Hui-cheng, had started out as an obscure Manchu official who worked as a clerk, a junior mandarin in the Board of Civil Appointments in Peking.

Hui-cheng had not been rich, therefore he was probably an honest man.[1] Little Orchid herself noted that she had not been "the favourite" with her family, and although she had been a real beauty* she didn't fit the standard Chinese idea of attractiveness. Little Orchid was short for a Manchu, just 1.5 metres tall. She had big black eyes, wing-like eyebrows, a broad high forehead, and a rounded chin. But her silky black hair, which she never cut, was a source of great pride. She was also one of the very few of her time to escape the ravages of both smallpox and goitre. Unlike *Han* Chinese women, Little Orchid had "big feet," because Manchu women had never bound their feet to produce the 7.5 centimetres "golden lilies" that Chinese men found so sexually stimulating. Throughout her life the Empress wore traditional Manchu shoes, rather like bejewelled clogs, that raised her to a lofty 1.7 metres.

On the third month of the moon year, the 208th year of Manchu rule in China,[2] Little Orchid and her cousin Sakota, or Niuhuru, as suitable daughters

*A painting of Tz'u-hsi at age 26 shows that she was really quite attractive in her youth, but she did not age gracefully.

of the ruling classes, had been summoned to appear at the Imperial Court. The girls were both about 17 years old. The 20 year-old Son of Heaven, the new Emperor Hsien-feng (of Universal Plenty), was choosing his harem for the day when the mourning period for his father, the Tao-kuang Emperor, would be over. Only two of 60 eligible Manchu girls, Little Orchid and Sakota had been dressed in the finest robes and jewels their somewhat impoverished family could borrow.

Seated cross-legged in closed sedan chairs, the young women had passed through the Wu Men (Gate of the Zenith), into the magnificent marble-and-tile Forbidden City. Rather than be presented to the Son of Heaven himself, they were paraded in front of the Emperor's stepmother, who was accompanied by the chief eunuch, An Teh-hai. The prospective concubines first were inspected for blemishes, defects and illness, questioned in Chinese and Manchu, and then examined in some elementary passages of the classics. Finally the five lucky characters of Little Orchid's birth ascertained that she, among a number of others, would be a suitable concubine for the Emperor. Hsien-feng himself was not even present at the selection.

Being a concubine did not guarantee access to the Chinese Emperor — some of these women spent their entire lives cloistered in their apartments without ever having met the exalted one, let alone having the honour of sharing his bed. Depending on how one looked at it, both Sakota and Little Orchid were the luckiest ones. On June 14, 1852, Sakota, whose deceased sister had been the wife of the Emperor,[3] was given the first rank of *Fei*, or First Imperial Concubine. Little Orchid was appointed only to third rank of *Kuei Jen*. She was now known as Yehonala, the name of her clansmen, and alternatively, Concubine Yi.

Life in the Forbidden City was incredibly organized, and thoroughly corrupt. Imperial boards, all run by the palace eunuchs, supervised vaults of gold and silver, furs, precious porcelains, silks and teas. Others controlled herds and flocks, butteries and kitchens. There were schools for Imperial offspring and even a police bureau. The spending was phenomenal. Sumptuous tributary gifts that poured in from China's vast provinces often rendered the sender bankrupt.

Yehonala was surrounded with eunuchs and seemed to enjoy their company more than that of her sister concubines. Perhaps because she was a strong character, the lack of threat posed by these high-voiced courtiers allowed her to become closer to men than she might otherwise have been allowed in 19th-century China. The eunuchs themselves were a strange lot — recruited into the palace by various princes for about $150 each. Although this was a lot of money for some, it would hardly seem worth emasculating oneself for this kind of fee.*

*Many eunuchs had also been sold by their families.

But the abject squalor that existed for all but a few of China's millions was obviously less attractive for these men. Entry to the Forbidden City promised riches, fine clothing, endless access to good food and, most important, a cut of all the money that passed through one's hands. The size of the cut depended on the cunning of the eunuch, and cunning guaranteed almost unlimited power.

Noted in her own remembrances, Yehonala had been bored stiff living in a harem, and because she had, at home, been allowed to learn how to read, she attached herself to an elderly scholar with whom she honed her reading, writing and her political skills. By studying Confucius and Mencius, the young concubine learned a great deal, not only of China's history but of Heaven as it related to the Imperial family. Confucian philosophy deemed that a benevolent ruler used solicitude and moral suasion, rather than force, to look after the welfare of his subjects. However, Confucius reasoned that a sense of discipline is necessary to maintain tranquillity and order. Like so many other philosophies and religions that fell into the same trap over the centuries, harmony had given way to ambitiousness, and benevolent rule had become a nebulous thread in a tangled mass of political scheming.

If one is going to take on an enormous task, and Yehonala was well on her way, one had better get it right. The studious concubine first plunged into *The Book of Filial Piety*, the tome that ruled Chinese society. In China the family was all — and respect for parents more important than life itself. When the

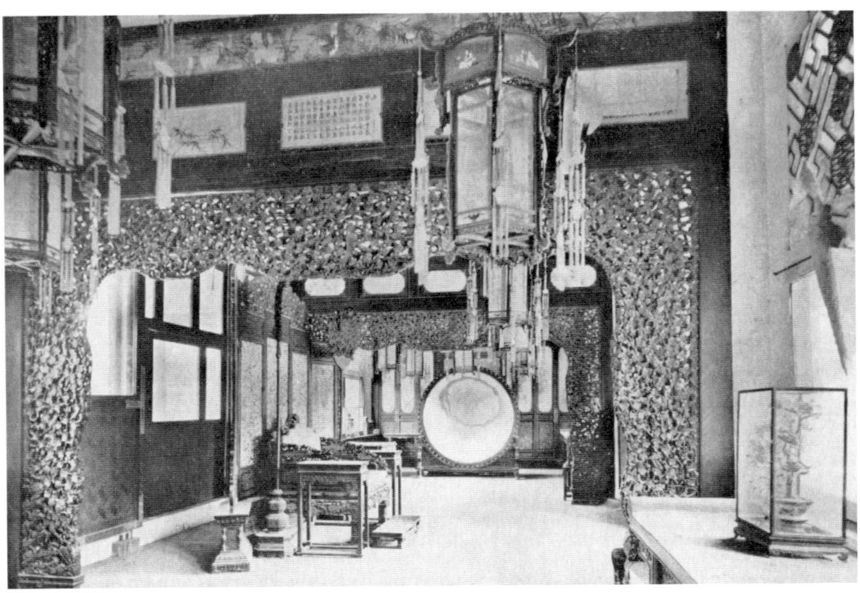

Tz'u-hsi's apartment

parents had gone the children carried on, and ancestor-worship dominated each day of their lives. Filial piety started out at the very centre of the Middle Kingdom, and that centre was the Son of Heaven, the Emperor himself. The ripples created by the Auspicious One naturally were strongest near the source and became weaker the farther away one moved on the pond. One could, even without noble birth, become a wavelet lapping right up against the source of power. Thus Yehonala, or Concubine Yi, improved herself by studying the gentle and admired arts of painting and calligraphy, manners and conversation. It was rumoured that she also managed to get hold of some forbidden erotica from the "men's library," but this seems unlikely.

Perhaps because he sensed greatness in the making, a young eunuch named Li Lien-ying attached himself to Yehonala, and maybe through successful planning on both their parts she was quickly brought to the attention of the Emperor and subsequently shared his bed. In comparison with delicate, weak-willed Niuhuru, Yehonala was strong and wilful, but she had also cultivated an exquisite courtesy and developed a quick mind that could read her Lord's moods and needs. As a matter of course she hid her physical disgust for the sickly and often impotent Emperor. This confused young man, tired of constant court intrigue and responsibility, had become increasingly decadent in his

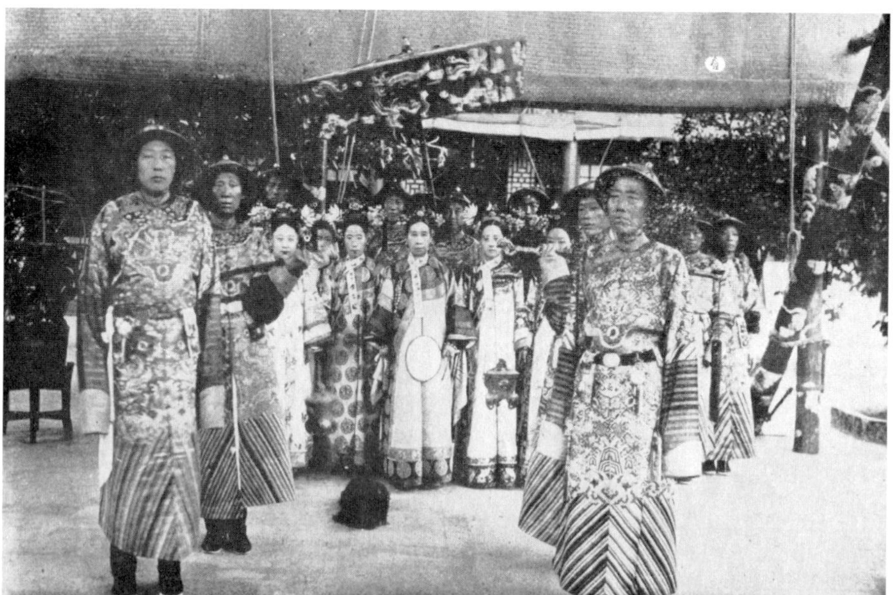

Tz'u-hsi, with the consort (Lung Yü) and principal concubine (Jen Fei) of Emperor Kuang-Hsü, accompanied by court ladies and eunuchs

behaviour, visiting sordid "flower boats" to taste the forbidden fruit of lily-footed Han Chinese whores, and cavorting in all manner with his eunuchs. It has been said that Hsien-feng drank copiously and smoked opium until he was incapable of telling the difference between boys and girls.

But obviously the Emperor was still capable of something, because Concubine Yi conceived in 1856 and was raised one level, to *Pin*. Shortly thereafter she gave birth to the son of the Emperor and heir to the throne. Reeling with joy, the Emperor had Yehonala promoted to the rank of Consort, equal to her cousin Niuhuru, the Empress Consort. To avoid confusion, Yehonala was called Tz'u-hsi, or Empress of the Western Palace, while Sakota was named Tz'u-an, Empress of the Eastern Palace. These two women, as different as night and day, would jointly rule the Middle Kingdom for many years to come.

Endnotes

1. Warner, Marina. *The Dragon Empress: Life and Times of Tz'u-hsi, 1835-1908, Empress Dowager of China*. London: Cardinal, 1974, p. 15.
2. Buck, Pearl S. *Imperial Woman*. New York: Pocket Cardinal edition, Pocket Books, Inc., 1964, p. 1.
3. Sakota's elder sister died an early death in the Forbidden City.

Chapter nine

The foreigners
1842–1870

Officers and men ... were absorbed in one pursuit ... plunder, plunder.
— Lord Elgin

The founder of medical missions in China was Dr. Peter Parker, an American who had opened an ophthalmic hospital in Canton on November 4, 1835. Because many Chinese suffered from cataracts and other eye complaints, Parker's hospital became a popular attraction and quickly grew into a general hospital and dispensary. Dr. Parker's favourite expression was that he was "opening China at the point of a lancet."* The interest in Western medicine, particularly surgical techniques, soon became widespread, and a number of young Chinese men began studying English with a view to gaining positions at the hospital. In 1838, to support the work, Parker established the Medical Missionary Society in China. It was this body that encouraged physicians to travel to China. Ultimately, if indirectly, Dr. Peter Parker was responsible for Leonora's arrival in 1877.

In 1842, Britain had declared war on China, asserting that if Chinese pirates could smuggle opium into the country, so too should they be allowed, and legally. Up to the infamous time of the Opium War, Western commerce had been confined to Canton and the Portuguese colony of Macao. The result of the Opium War was the opening of the five ports of Canton, Amoy, Foochow, Ningpo and Shanghai to foreign trade, and to foreign residence. No matter that millions would die from addiction and its related evils, even the most well-meaning missionaries found an excuse for the barbarous enterprise.

In his *Forty Years in China*, for instance, Reverend R.H. Graves wrote that "War ... is like a cyclone that spreads devastation in its path ... but purifying the

*A lancet is a small, broad, two-edged surgical knife.

atmosphere, and making life possible removing the germs of disease and death." God, he said, often accomplished His beneficent purposes by violent means. The Opium Wars of 1842, he noted, though morally unjustifiable, proved the "entering wedge ... and ... when an opening is made, the good and bad flow in together."[1]

While young Tz'u-hsi was rising to fame in the Forbidden City, the Westerners in their treaty ports were again itching to expand their Chinese holdings. They had easily managed to convince themselves that free trade (plus a bit of Christianity) would equal civilization. Four hundred million Chinese were, they believed, just waiting to get their hands on foreign goods, particularly opium. The religious societies knew that 400 million souls would, in turn, need to be saved. A neat partnership began to form between merchant and missionary.

Just after Tz'u-hsi had given birth to the heir to the throne, a Hong Kong ship, the *Arrow*, was boarded by Chinese officers who arrested the crew for piracy and pulled down the British flag she was flying. It was 1856. The ship's English captain rapidly related the insult to Harry Parkes, Britain's Consul in Canton. Parkes, who had a reputation of treating the Chinese with incredible incivility, stridently demanded an apology and the freedom of three crew suspected of piracy. Commissioner Yeh Ming-ch'en refused. Although he did not know it at the time, he was right to do so, because the *Arrow*'s Hong Kong registration had expired, and she was no longer entitled to fly the British flag.

By October 27, the British had seized the forts at the entrance of Canton harbour, and Yeh was being bombarded by British cannon. The French, fed on a gory tale of a missionary death and dismemberment, joined forces with the British. After the Opium Wars of 1842, the British public had wanted no further conflict with China, but finally the government prevailed, sending Lord Elgin, a former Governor General of Canada, as the British Envoy. His job was to demand reparation in the form of cash indemnity and far greater freedom for the foreign community in China. If not granted, Elgin declared he would use force to ensure British representation in the hitherto "closed" city of Peking. This was good news for merchant and missionary alike, because both groups were chafing to move ever farther into this rich and exotic land.

But in order to understand Chinese resistance to foreign influences, we need again to look at the *Arrow* affair of 1856. Just prior to the incident, a Hakka peasant named Hung Hsiu-chu'an had decided, after a vivid dream, that he was the brother of Jesus Christ and that he had a mission to redeem the oppressed, which his Hakka people most certainly were. Indeed he "wandered in the wilderness," making thousands of converts. His radical ideas of reform included making all monies public, to be shared by the whole populace. Obviously, this did not sit well with the vastly wealthy Manchus, or even with their Han Chinese officials. Thus began what became known as the Taiping Rebellion.

Hung had started off with the best intentions. By March 1853, he had gained an army of 250,000 and captured Nanking, the most prestigious city in southern China. Here the Heavenly King, as he described himself, forbade fortune-telling and soothsaying, tobacco, alcohol and opium. He segregated women from men and declared that men who hired women to cook and sew for them would be executed. Polygamy and prostitution were banned, and adultery was punished severely.

But just after this period, Hung Hsiu-chu'an fell into the almost inevitable abyss of despotism. As Heavenly King, he chose trusted disciples and named them kings of the North, South and West (presumably he was the Eastern King), and he even named an assistant king, rather like a deputy prime minister or a vice-president. Now he began to array himself in the forbidden Manchu imperial yellow silks, and the chosen few followed suit. Hung, who eventually claimed 88 wives, sent a message to Peking that he was to be known as the Lord of Ten Thousand Years, a title reserved for the Manchu Emperor. The illustrious general Tseng Kuo-fan hired a youthful soldier, Li Hung-chang, to quell the rebels. A band of Shanghai irregulars, led by American Frederick Ward, soon became a 4,000-strong Chinese force called "The Ever-Victorious Army." Li Hung-chang, almost unique among Chinese who trusted foreigners, eventually took over, asking the British for one of their best soldiers. Charles George Gordon, "Chinese Gordon" and "Gordon of Khartoum," besieged Nanking, where "Heavenly King" Hung dispensed pearls rather than food. On June 30, Hung committed suicide. Gordon was awarded, on the advice of Li Hung-chang, the Yellow Riding Jacket, similar to being made a knight of the garter in Britain.

To make a long story short, the British, still seething over the *Arrow* affair, found that Hung's Taiping rebels might be just the ticket to aid and abet their own plans for the Middle Kingdom. The French joined the British in their condemnation of the Manchu throne.

In May 1858, the French and English, who had moved their gunboats up as far as Tientsin, attacked the Taku Forts, heretofore believed impregnable because of the wide Pei Ho River and miles of salt flats and dangerous marshland. By June the Chinese, tired from the Taiping Rebellion, buckled to the foreigners' demands and signed more of their land in what became known as the Treaty of Tientsin. But there remained one more bone of contention: even the Americans, who had acted as impartial observers throughout the disturbances, refused to kowtow before the Emperor. The British and the French issued an ultimatum, including demands for indemnities, for apologies, and for expanding the foreign "residence" treaty of Shanghai. The Chinese prevaricated, thinking that maybe if this nuisance were ignored, it would go away. But by August 21, 1860, the Taku Forts at Tientsin had surrendered to the foreigners.

The most shameful behaviour now began on both sides. Having left a great deal of death and destruction in their wakes, Harry Parkes and his associate, Henry Loch, spiked a white handkerchief on a lance as a sign of truce. A Mongol officer by the name of Seng-ko-lin-ch'in claimed them as prisoners and marched them, bound on poles, to Peking and the vilest of prisons. Another battle broke out and 13 English and French were taken prisoner, then "barbarously murdered."[2] On September 29, Parkes and Loch were transferred, courtesy of Tz'u-hsi's highest adviser, Prince Kung, to better quarters, although they were still not released. By October, French and English forces had converged upon Tz'u-hsi's most beloved place of rest, the Summer Palace. The French General assured the British that he had forbidden looting, but the knowledge of magnificent treasures, golden statues, fabulous jewels and jade fountains led to an orgy of destruction. Even the British chaplain, Reverend McGhee, accompanied a friend in the frenzy and reported that he had a wonderful time. Finally, nothing remained of the ancient and magnificent complex of palaces and temples, but smoke, rubble and the outline of a "European" palace, modelled on Versailles, that had been designed by the Jesuits in the preceding century. China, if not entirely vanquished, was simply pushed into submission by superior arms.

By the time Leonora set foot in The Middle Kingdom, both the Emperor and his youthful heir had died — Hsien Feng from his profligate habits and Tz'u-hsi's cherished son T'ung Chih (of Pervading Peace) to smallpox before his 20th birthday. It has been written that T'ung Chih had already, like his own father, been weakened by unseemly behaviour and suffered from venereal disease. Like his father, he had drunk copiously and used more opium than was good for him. Whether or not this is true, the northern Chinese were, on the whole, remarkably resistant to dying from smallpox. Emperor T'ung Chih had indeed rallied for a few months, but was felled by recurring fever on January 12, 1875. He had been married for three years to a beautiful and strong-willed noblewoman called Alute. Perhaps because she herself had not produced an heir, or perhaps horrified at the thought of spending her life kowtowing to mother-in-law Tz'u-hsi, Alute committed suicide just 74 days after the Emperor's death. Tz'u-hsi immediately proclaimed that her nephew, three-year-old Tsai-t'ien, would be sworn in as the Kuang-hsu Emperor — of glorious succession — on February 25, 1875. Tz'u-hsi and her cousin Niuhuru effectively ruled the Middle Kingdom.

By 1870, the Westerners had gained a strong foothold in the treaty port of Tientsin, just 120 kilometres from Peking. They were not, however, very popular. A Crown lease had been signed as part of the Conventions of Peking in 1860 and Anglo-French troops remained at the Taku Forts. In addition, the French had seized an imperial villa to use as a consulate. By 1863 English missionary John Innocent had saved enough silver to purchase land on which to build a bungalow, a warehouse, a business office, and a hotel. The earliest Astor Hotel was known as "Mud House" (Ni Wu) and "Old House" (Lao Wu). This was, in fact, the origin of the "British Concession."

In 1869, the church and orphanage of Notre Dame des Victoires was constructed on the site of a razed Buddhist temple. Orphans seemed to be at a premium, because few Chinese would entrust them to foreigners. The nuns, therefore, offered silver for each child, thus encouraging unscrupulous child brokers to kidnap the little ones. This, plus the fact nuns were particularly interested in baptizing sick and dying children, led to rumours that they bewitched the children, mutilated their bodies, and extracted hearts and eyes to make medicines. For many years hence, Leonora would have to battle rumours that her treatments would kill the patients.

One year after the orphanage had opened, Ch'ung-hou, superintendent of trade for northern ports, inspected the premises and proclaimed to a large mob there was no truth to the rumours. Unfortunately for all concerned, the French consul, Henri Fontanier, appeared with his assistant, demanding justice. Fontanier fired a shot that missed Ch'ung-hou, but killed his manservant. In retaliation, the mob killed the Frenchman and his assistant, then set fire to the church and orphanage. In what became known in the West as the "Tientsin Massacre," 10 nuns, two priests, two French officials and three Russian traders were killed, and four British and American churches were destroyed.

Tz'u-hsi appointed Tseng Kuo-fan, by now Viceroy of Chihli Province, to investigate. Highly intelligent and widely respected, he agreed that Britain, the United States and Russia be indemnified first to disassociate themselves from the French cause. He learned first hand from the Chinese orphans that they had not been kidnapped at all, and that any "eyes" being displayed to the crowds had been jars of preserved cherries. He asked the court at Peking to issue a proclamation denying the rumours of ill-treatment by the nuns. Tseng then recommended dismissing the Tientsin prefect and district magistrate, executing 15 of the instigators of the riot and banishing 21 others. This quest for justice was cause for outrage among Chinese conservative scholars in Peking, who subsequently burned Tseng's revered poetry. Li Hung-chang, by now Viceroy of Wuchang, suggested that only eight instigators be executed, and 20 exiled. Tseng was transferred to Nanking, and Li entered his finest hour as Viceroy of Chihli Province. He would reside in a magnificent palace in Tientsin, and it would be in this very abode that Leonora Howard's own destiny would unfold some six years later.

Endnotes

1. Graves, R.H., D.D. *Forty Years in China or China in Transition*. Baltimore, Maryland: R.H. Woodward Company, 1895, pp. 118-119.
2. Warner, Marina. *The Dragon Empress: Life and Times of Tz'u-hsi, 1835-1908, Empress Dowager of China*. London: Cardinal, 1974, pp. 65-69.

Chapter ten

The Peking district
1878

Thou shalt have no other gods before me.
— Exodus 20:3

If Leonora had hoped for instant conversions to Christianity, she was quickly put to rights by the alternate indifference and hostility of the Chinese. To add insult to injury, she, like most newcomers, would soon become ill, then anemic and subject to constant low fevers for the rest of her life. Mixed emotions also took their toll. Many without an almost fanatic belief in "the cause" gradually became disenchanted and, subsequently, wracked with guilt that they had somehow failed in the Lord's work. But in a sense Leonora was luckier than most. It was soon apparent that floods, famine and disease would keep her far too busy to bother with religious frustrations.

But frustrating it was. In 1879, Chester Holcombe of the London Missionary Society wrote that it was "hard to convince Chinamen that to enter the religion is not to entitle themselves to a fair share, perhaps to a Lion's Share, of the distribution. ... in the places where famine relief has actually taken place, the natives one and all have an opportunity of seeing that *distress*, not *religion* is the ground of the relief, that Christians who are not in distress do not get it, and that heathens who are in distress do get it." Therein lay quite a dilemma.

There was also a dawning sense of horror that it would take years to make even one or two converts, and that these were usually outcasts from their families or society at large. These "Rice Christians" readily accepted the Western God in return for a hot meal, and many converted to two or three different creeds in the space of a week. Sometimes the Westerners' only reward was the knowledge that those at home would talk of their self-sacrifice after their (often speedy) demise. Many who survived to become Old China Hands became superbly cynical, doctoring conversion figures to appease the Boards back home and to justify requests for funding. Who would be the wiser? Still others became victims of internal politics. Squabbling over accommodations, in particular, became an escape valve for a lot of pent-up anger.

After many letters to and fro, these squabbles often became official "cases." One such was "The Quest of Dr. Dudgeon's Drug Room and Study", where the party of the first part complained that while he was away, his drug room was seized, "my drugs, valuable books ... many instruments ... etc. were moved into a locked room ... many of my drugs and medical stores are scattered over the compound or left unpacked standing in courtyards." Dr. Dudgeon's nemesis was a new arrival, Mr. Gilmour. Gilmour's wife apparently decided that she and her husband had precedence over Dudgeon's absence but, Dr. Dudgeon insisted, Gilmour had "never breathed a syllable of any desire on his part or that of his wife to possess my drug room ... ." This particular portion of the argument raged on for 45 closely written pages,[1] and the "case" itself took almost a year to resolve. Thus was deflected a great deal of disappointment in the brutal realities of missionary work in China, and thus also was boredom averted.

Because of the fear of riots, new female recruits were often confined to the deadly routine of the mission compound. Their only exercise might be a daily walk on top of the compound wall, well away from hostile villagers. Later on, Canadian women at the China Inland Mission would send home reports about their exercise in the yard, walking, skipping and most often, playing tennis. This became known as the "missionaries' game" because it was one of the few healthy activities open to everyone. Tennis would eventually catch on with China's last Emperor, Pu Yi himself. Neither his Manchu Empress nor his concubine had bound feet, and trapped in the Forbidden City as surely as the missionary women were trapped in the compounds, they would all play the game with gusto.

Missionaries living in, or travelling to, the Chinese interior, frequently adopted Chinese dress to appear less obtrusive, and also to prevent the inevitable staring, handling and pulling of clothing that all Westerners encountered. Some of the men went to the extent of growing queues and shaving their foreheads, as was the Chinese fashion of the time. The best-laid plans frequently backfired, however, when missionaries who dressed in one village fashion ventured into another area where the clothing, even the mode of transportation, was markedly different, and therefore suspect. As one woman remarked on her travels "I had, as I thought, eschewed all foreign articles of attire, going bare-headed and looking as much like a Chinese woman as big nose, big feet, and light hair would permit, but still my long robe of fine cotton cloth ... and my umbrella now and then proved more interesting than the difference between the true God and the temple idols."[2]

Female missionaries in China's interior were given a type of fashion freedom not afforded Leonora, residing in the great capital of Peking. One woman wrote that although her blue sateen dress was old fashioned, she lived in blissful ignorance of what was stylish, and it did not affect her happiness at all. Another expressed her relief from fashion's tyranny by writing, "... Mama, you would like the restfulness of our life ... I don't mean that we work less than at home ... but then there isn't *any* worry about styles or hats or anything until the last thread is gone."[3]

But the inland missionaries were aghast at what was expected when they visited the big city. One young woman wrote "I suspect you think this sounds rather foxy for a missionary ... but ... from the clothes standpoint, living in Peking is no joke ... it's not just a matter of wanting to be in fashion; it's necessary if we and our work are to be respected [by colonial society]." Other members of the WFMS wrote different types of letters to different audiences. Writing to Mother at home, one might ask offhandedly for "stray fashion sheets" so as not to become "too antiquated." To a colleague, one woman on furlough reported that although she had wanted an elegant gown made in Paris, she had had her China silk made up in London. "You will groan, for London isn't considered a stylish place, but it isn't half bad." Another went on to describe the latest "swell" party gown, of "Chinese gauze, white or black, for a half length skirt, some chiffon to mix in with the waist, and the rest white or delicate colored plain silk or satin. Brocades in big figures are stylish too."[4]

During this time, cotton goods from Manchester, were exported by the ton to what was supposed to be an eager Chinese consumer. In fact, English cotton was universally sneered at for its poor cut and quality. The British cloth, it was agreed, was the wrong width for Chinese clothing — some 20 centimetres was wasted after it was cut. In addition, the cloth and its wrappers were constantly displaying colours that were unlucky in China. Printed cottons, besides being offensive in colour, were considered coarse in pattern, colouring and style. Quite simply the Chinese did not want these goods at any price. Where a rich Western consumer might throw away last year's garments in the name of fashion, those garments would in any case last only one quarter as long as the good, strong, hand-woven items available in the Middle Kingdom. Even when a coolies' clothes were worn to rags, the cloth was still good for other purposes. Finally, British products were said to be far too thin for winter wear: the Chinese product was twice the weight.

Over her Western wool dresses, Leonora would probably have worn padded Chinese cotton coats in winter. The blazing heat of summer demanded cool dimity cottons and fine, breathable, Chinese silks. Her professional wear was a long dark dress with a trim white collar. An ungainly pith helmet which was, in reality, "very light and cool; at any rate we must put looks aside and wear it," was de rigueur in the field. She may indeed, like some other women, have improved the pith helmet's appearance by having embroidered covers made for the hats.

But fashion aside, missionary doctors and nurses were a breed apart from run-of-the-mill evangelists, measuring their success not so much in souls saved as in bodies healed, diseases conquered, and hospitals built. In fact, doctors of all missionary societies found they had less and less time for evangelizing. In 1877, the year of Leonora's arrival, Dr. William Gauld warned his colleagues at the Shanghai Missionary Conference not to let "philanthropic and scientific aspects engross our whole mind and strength."[5]

In this, her first year, Leonora learned that the Chinese did recognize a supreme God of sorts (*Shangtien hou*) and a hereafter, or merit place, hence the importance given to good behaviour and ancestor worship. When the Muslims had settled in China, they could not quite reconcile the Confucian idea of a god, so they named theirs (*Chen Chu*) for "True Lord." The Jesuits could not recognize either of these gods, and initially named their god *Shang ti*, or "Supreme Ruler," which didn't sit too well with the various Emperors. The priests subsequently changed the Chinese characters to read *Tien Chu*, or "Lord of Heaven," which was a little more appropriate. As a Methodist, Leonora naturally could not be identified with the Roman Catholics, and she would have been told to use *Chen Shen* for "the true Spirit," thereby suggesting that the other spirits might be false.[6] What made matters worse for those few Chinese interested in the Western religion was that in 1884, a Dr. Blodget of Peking rejected most of the existing terms and decided that the Jesuits' *Tien Chu* (Lord of Heaven) would better serve the missionaries' cause. It was little wonder that Leonora's patients, who were used to worshipping many spirits, became totally confused when her Bible Women — usually Chinese converts — kept insisting that there was only one true God, and this was His latest name.

Apart from the religious obstacle, Leonora's most formidable opponent was the Chinese pharmacist. An amazing variety of herbs and animal-based drugs were available in the average Chinese pharmacopoeia. Among the most upsetting for some Western animal lovers was the sight of a live stag tethered behind the shop awaiting sure doom. "Pills manufactured out of a whole stag slaughtered with purity of purpose on a propitious day," was a common announcement posted at these dispensaries. Also, "from the bones of leopards, an admirable tonic may be distilled," and that prepared from tiger bones was the greatest of all, conferring the courage and strength of the animal upon the drinker.

Examinations offered by Chinese pharmacists, or "doctors," largely consisted of feeling the many and varied pulses of their patients. Among, for example, the seven kinds of pulse said to presage death, were the following:

1. When the pulse is perceived under the fingers to bubble irregularly like water over a great fire, if it be in the morning, the patient will die in the evening.
2. Death is no farther off if the pulse seems like a fish whose head is stopped in such a manner that he cannot move, but has a risking tail without any regularity; the cause of this distemper lies in the kidneys.
3. If the pulse seems like drops of water that fall into a room through some crack, and when it is returned it is scattered and disordered much like the twine of a cord which is unravelled, the bones are dried up even to the very marrow.
4. If the motion ... resembles the pace of a frog when he is embarrassed in the weeds, death is certain.
5. If the motion ... resembles the hasty pecking of the beak of a bird, there is a defect in the spirits of the stomach.[7]

Medicines operated according to their taste on the tongue. Sour medicines were to "impede or retain," bitter ones to cause "looseness and warmth as well as hardening," sweet to "strengthen, harmonize and warm," acid to "disperse, prove emollient, and go in an athwart direction," salt would help matters to "descend," and those substances that were hard and tasteless would "open the orifices and promote a discharge." Appeasing the gods was easy for those afflicted with ague (rheumatism). All the patient had to do was write the names of the eight demons of ague on paper, then eat the paper (with cake), or presumably if not literate, to take the eyes out of one's neighbour's paper door-god. Eating these, said the pharmacists, guaranteed a cure. If it didn't work, well, the patient must have angered her ancestors or have been born on an unlucky day. And there was nothing they could do about *that*.

As a rule, the Chinese did not like to be touched unless the person doing the touching knew them very well. Traditional herbalists would attempt cures more by asking questions than by touching a patient's body. Leonora's Western medical practices would certainly have terrified the less educated of her patients. Indeed, much of the rumour concerning the "Foreign Devils" revolved around what the Chinese assumed were normal western medical practices. The idea that they plucked out the eyes of Chinese children for use in alchemy and medicine may be traced back as far as 1660[8] and to the funeral rites of the Roman Catholic Church. Here the Chinese would see priests performing "magical incantations" of sprinkling holy water, then covering the face with a cloth. According to rumour, the priest, while pretending to pray, would then extract the eyes and replace them with coins. The most common evidence of this would by the dramatic production of a jar of preserved cherries — obviously the stolen eyes.

But the biggest problem in China remained the terrible lack of sanitation. Unfortunately some Chinese doctors tended to assure their patients that if human excrement were no longer allowed to accumulate in the streets, "where it might attract the putrescent particles floating in the air," these noxious vapours might enter the body and pestilential sickness would inevitably result. In the southerly, coastal districts, the bubonic plague and cholera reared their monstrous heads with alarming regularity. Smallpox, known as "Heavenly Flowers" was alternately a terrible scourge in western China or a badge of honour among the northerners, who seemed to come through the disease fairly well. Dr. George Morrison, an Australian adventurer who became the Peking correspondent for the *Times*, related that inoculation was practised by introducing a dried pock-scab, on a lucky day, into one of the patient's nostrils. This preventive didn't seem to work too often, though, because whole villages lined up to be inoculated when news of Leonora's western vaccine spread through Chihli Province.

Finally there would be some opposition from Leonora's own colleagues in the field. Fundamentalists like Jonathan Goforth, the first official Canadian missionary in China, would not help her cause for improved medical practices. A firm believer in "Divine Healing," he himself almost died from pneumonia. Refusing to take any medicine and forbidding his wife to call a doctor, he grew steadily worse. Mrs. Goforth finally ignored his commands, calling in Dr. James Menzies, who prescribed quinine. Within a week, Goforth was back on his feet, but the treatment did not, Menzies related, destroy the preacher's belief in Divine Healing.

Another Canadian, Dr. Robert McClure, wrote that "The big problem in the early days of medicine in China really was how scientific you would be. This was an ethical problem with the individual doctor and it was always a struggle. For instance, every time you raised your standards, you raised the cost and therefore the price to the patient. As (modern) medicine came into China, you first of all had antiseptic medicine ... The sterilized sheet, the drapes ... Then as antiseptic medicine was accepted ... and rapidly followed by sterile techniques and scrubbed hands ... you had this tremendous struggle."

Roman Catholic missions addressed the problem by never going into modern medicine at all. The Grey Sisters from Pembroke, Ontario, working in Chekian, handed out quinine tablets and worm pills, and the Missionary Sisters of the Immaculate Conception ran leprosaria in Canton and Manchuria, and that was about it. But Protestants like Leonora used the most modern methods available, particularly surgical techniques like removing cataracts, although she did not, like other missionaries, charge for her services.

Home board policy had repeatedly stated that hospitals and clinics should meet the highest standards, and she took these orders quite seriously. Although a later Canadian Methodist report stated that "unsanitary hospitals are a reproach to Western medical science and to Christianity," doctors like Leonora had great difficulty incorporating modern ways into traditional Chinese lifestyles. Her battle would go on well into the 20th century.

Endnotes

1. Council for World Missionary Archives, Day Missions Library, Yale University. London Missionary Society Reports. Box H-2139. 1879.
2. Hunter, Jane. *The Gospel of Gentility - American Women Missionaries in Turn-of-the-Century China*. New Haven: Yale University Press, 1984, p. 19.
3. Ibid., pp. 135-136.
4. Ibid., p. 137.
5. Liu, Kwang-Ching, ed. *American Missionaries in China*. Cambridge, Mass.: East Asian Research Center, Harvard University Press, 1970, p. 107.
6. Morrison, G.E. (Chinese). *An Australian in China*. Sydney, Australia: Angus and Robertson Pty Ltd., 1972, pp. 122-123.
7. Ibid., p. 108.
8. Austin, Alvyn J. *Saving China: Canadian Missionaries in the Middle Kingdom, 1888-1959*. Toronto: University of Toronto Press, 1986, p. 74.

Chapter eleven

Lady Li's cure
1879

"You can see how the matter stands."
— Leonora Howard, MD

Viceroy Tseng Kuo-fan had died in Nanking in 1873. Tseng's former military colleague, Li Hung-chang, had replaced him as Viceroy of Chihli province in the aftermath of the tragic Tientsin massacre. Li, who had risen through the ranks, was remarkably interested in Western technology. This was not to say he was pro-Western, but he simply wanted to create a China that could hold its own against foreign invasion. So Li Hung-chang plunged into modernization with as much enthusiasm as his regal post would allow, and in the process he gained respect for Western medicine.

Li was a huge man, almost 2 metres tall. Although of less than noble birth,* he had a patrician face and over the years had developed a dignified demeanour. As the highest-ranked Viceroy in the Middle Kingdom, Li wore a round black hat with a red crown and precious ruby mandarin's button held in place with a peacock's feather. Unlike some more flamboyant mandarins, he usually dressed in rich, heavy, light blue and grey silks. In winter he might wear a red-and-purple striped underskirt, reminiscent of the Empress Dowager's favourite yellow-and-purple garments, but it was, for the main, covered by a black satin overdress and rich sable coat.† Li Hung-chang generally dispensed with the thick ropes of pearl, precious jade or coral that even the "Foreign Mandarin," British General Charles Gordon, wore with great flash and bravura. The formidable Li had a moustache and beard that could rival many of the

*China, more than any place in the world, relied more on the "merit principle" for elevating her subjects, rather than nobility by birth.

†The only people allowed to wear sable were given this singular right by the Emperor. Sable signified great favour and mandarin status.

Westerners' own elegant whiskers. His fiery black almond eyes could reduce lesser mortals to a state of terror, but for his own family he had, for the times, a curious soft spot. Greying now in middle age, he projected power and wealth. Li Hung-chang was not someone you would wish to argue with.

Li was now a veteran politician. In 1865, the Empress Dowager had appointed him acting viceroy of Liang-kiang. In 1867, he was named viceroy of Hunan and Hupeh and, finally, in 1871, she had given him the coveted viceroyalty of Chihli Province. Almost immediately Li moved the provincial capital from the small town of Paoting to the port of Tientsin, where he would have more contact with the foreign powers. It was here, rather than Paoting, that Li would choose to honour his predecessor, Tseng Kuo-fan. Because Tseng had lived such a pure Confucian life, Empress Dowager Tz'u-hsi had decreed that memorial temples should be built in his honour in each province. Li constructed a fine green-and-gold temple, just outside his own yamen, or vice-regal palace. This temple would in a very short time change Leonora's life forever.

Li Hung-chang had invested heavily in things modern, including the Western-style hotel in the British Concession, the first railroad and telegraph lines to Peking, a lucrative coal mine, and a vast merchant shipping line. There are varying reports of Li's corruption versus his diplomatic greatness, but it is probably fair to say that regarding the former, he was no better and no worse than any Chinese official of the times. Regarding the latter, he has gone down in history as the period's most important statesmen.

In his own way, Dr. John Kenneth Mackenzie of the London Missionary Society (LMS) was also very prominent. In China since 1875, he had lived for a time in Hankow, serving in a hospital erected by the LMS and helped by the gifts of Chinese and foreign residents. Because of his wife's less than robust health, he had moved to the more favourable climes of Tientsin.[1] The record of Mackenzie's life seems, in many respects, a model for aspiring missionaries. As the *Chinese Recorder* noted, "Fervour and spirituality characterized his religious experience, and as a missionary physician he steadily kept in view the one cherished object of bringing recovery and health both to the souls and bodies of men." Writing of his own work in Hankow, Mackenzie said "my great aim is to make the hospital a means of proclaiming the Gospel and reaching the hearts of people through kindness and whatever benefits medically one can give them ... I make every serious operation a subject for prayer and I am thankful to God that no death has occurred, even after the most severe operations." Mackenzie was not alone in being grateful — most missionaries, including young Leonora, lived with the knowledge that death from an operation might very well result in their own decapitation.

Two years after Leonora's arrival, in summer of 1879, Li Hung-chang's wife fell seriously ill. It is not certain what was wrong with her, but it is likely she had a gynaecological problem. As John Kenneth Mackenzie and a Dr. Irwin were setting up a clinic in Tientsin, they were called to the vicereine's bedside. What followed has been reported in various forms by Mackenzie himself, Mackenzie's biographer, British missionary Mrs. Bryson, Leonora herself, and by the WFMS. Here is Mrs. Bryson's account of what occurred that spring. It was written in 1891, 12 years after the incident. Mrs. Bryson called this "the incident by which he [Mackenzie] became known to the outside world." It was certainly the incident by which Leonora became known throughout China, the United States, Canada and Europe.

> "Li Hung-chang, on the advice of a member of the British legation, had reluctantly sent for Drs. Irwin[2] and Mackenzie to attend Lady Li, who was thought to be dying. Accompanied by the Viceroy's private secretary,[3] they at once rode up to the Yamen. After an interview with His Excellency, who was deeply attached to his wife, and in her serious illness, had practically suspended all government business, they were conducted into the inner apartments of the sick lady. This, to Western ideas, would be a very natural and ordinary occurrence; but to Chinese notions it was a very extraordinary proceeding. 'Years ago,' noted Dr. Mackenzie, 'in Hangkow, I was called in to attend a sick lady, but I was not allowed to see her face. A hole was made in a curtain, through which her arm was protruded, that I might examine her pulse and so diagnose the disease. In this case we two foreign doctors had free permission to examine and question our patient, who was the wife of the leading Viceroy of the Empire.' They found the lady very ill—in a most critical condition, and at first did not seem to have been hopeful of a successful issue."*
>
> "It was necessary for Dr. Mackenzie to come down to the settlement for medicines and upon his return home he found a number of Christian natives in his colleague's study, earnestly talking over the wonderful event of the day. 'What chance was there of Lady Li's recovery?' was the eager enquiry from all; but the doctor could give no very hopeful reply. 'She is

*Because the word "issue" is used here, the author is assuming that Lady Li was in the process of giving birth to her son.

> very ill; I fear there is not much hope,' he said, 'but you must just keep on praying.'
>
> He returned to his illustrious patient and remained in the yamen all night, to enable the Viceroy, whose anxiety was now somewhat allayed, to get some needed sleep. 'We were in close attendance, seeing our patient twice a day for six days,' writes the doctor, 'when, by the mercy of God, the lady was, humanly speaking, out of danger.' Dr. Mackenzie's colleague well remembers how, on his return from the yamen, in reply to his interested enquiries about the case, he replied, 'Yes, she is recovering, she will do well now; but it is the result of no skill of mine, it is just God answering our prayers!'

The answer to Dr. Mackenzie's prayers then arrived in a slightly more human form — that of Dr. Leonora Howard. "It became necessary for the patient's complete restoration to health to adopt a certain line of treatment which, according to Chinese etiquette, could only be carried out by a lady. We therefore informed the Viceroy that at Peking (two days' journey off) there was an American [sic] lady doctor working in connection with the Methodist Episcopal Mission, Miss Howard, MD, and enquired if there would be any objection to a foreign lady carrying out our suggested treatment. 'None whatever!' was his reply."*

> "That day a special messenger was despatched to invite Miss Dr. Howard to come to Tientsin; the Viceroy, at the same time, sending his own steam launch to convey her from Tung-chow along the Pei Ho (river). Apartments within the Chinese palace were prepared for her, and here, upon the lady's arrival, she took up her abode, remaining in the yamen for a month, and was able to render invaluable assistance in the case."

Mackenzie added: "If you will try and realize the conditions of an Eastern city, you will quickly understand that when a great potentate takes you by the hand the land is all before you."

Thus began Leonora Howard's real tale, which read, wrote one woman at home, like a "story from *The Arabian Nights*."[4]

On being collected from Peking, Leonora would have been accompanied by at least one of her own senior servants, a nursing assistant, a translator

*It is difficult to imagine "none whatever!" emanating from a Chinese mandarin. This would have initially been Li's Secretary, Mr. Pethick's, interpretation, related to Mrs. Bryson by people who knew Dr. Mackenzie in past years. "None whatever!" in Chinese, would probably have taken about an hour to discuss.

(probably a missionary or Chinese Bible woman), a total of about 24 chair-bearers, and four of Li Hung-chang's outriders. This entourage was just to take her 2 or 3 kilometres to the canal, and thence to the Pei Ho River, where the crew of Li's sumptuous steam-launch awaited.

Up to now Leonora had never stepped foot in a Chinese home, with the exception of filthy village hovels, because Westerners, particularly women, were just not invited. But Li Hung-chang's palace was another matter entirely. Li had, as we have noted, already weighed the pros and cons of dealing with foreigners, and in this case the pro side clearly won the day. There was also, of course, the matter of delicacy. Lady Li must have sincerely welcomed a young female doctor, rather than the gruff bearded Englishmen who invaded her privacy.

Leonora would have been met by Li's American secretary, Mr. Pethick, at the gate, and led by servants through several courtyards full of brilliant azaleas, peonies, cherry blossoms and beautifully sculpted shrubs. The outer courtyard of the Viceroy's yamen would normally be filled with petitioners, lesser-ranked mandarins, servants and soldiers. But Li, in turmoil over his wife's illness, had suspended almost all government business and the outer courtyard was almost empty. As Leonora was led farther and farther into the huge palace complex, she must have marvelled at how the intricate carving of doors and rooftops could so beautifully complement the simple lines of shining brass censers, or incense burners, that perfumed the air against the rank odour of the city beyond. Now, in early summer, graceful willows leaned gently over jade-green ponds filled with creamy gold water lilies.

The heavy red doors opened as if by magic, beckoning her inside the main palace hall. Heels tapping on floors made of fine wood, the young doctor would enter a room decorated with priceless scrolls and silk paintings, some thousands of years old. Valuable polished blackwood chairs were as delicately carved as any temple roof. Inlaid into the back of each chair was a "marble landscape" with dark green markings that created restful scenes of water, mountains or forests. The furniture arrangement followed a strict traditional pattern. A long, exquisitely worked table was set against a wall facing the entry. On the table rested a pair of candles and a small incense urn. Between the candles hung a magnificent scroll commemorating Li Hung-chang's ancestors. In front was a smaller, square table with two high armchairs on each side. As a woman, Leonora would not be asked to take the chair on the right-hand side of the table. As a secondary "employee," and certainly not of any diplomatic rank, the doctor would be shown a chair at one of the smaller tables placed near enough so that she could speak and be heard. The least important guests, although today there were none, were always placed nearest the door.

Li Hung-chang would have offered the doctor delicate, exquisitely decorated porcelain cups of precious jasmine tea that was poured by a silent manservant. There were no women to be seen. By now Leonora would have learned that according to custom, she must accept the tea with both hands, then wait for her host to start the conversation. It would have been a serious breach of etiquette to interrupt the rhythm of this ceremony, even with Lady Li lying ill in her own quarters. As it was also unheard of for anyone to *appear* to see any woman who might pass through, the position in which Leonora found herself was peculiar indeed. Even when talking, the Viceroy would have to be particularly careful not to look at Leonora directly while speaking: looking a few inches above her head would, to the Chinese mind, prevent grave insult.

Leonora's first three weeks[5] in Tientsin were spent in her own, sumptuously decorated apartments, with more servants than she had ever seen. In the months that followed, when Lady Li and Leonora became fast friends, she would often be invited to the Vicereine's inner sanctum, which had its own graceful courtyards and was decorated to Lady Li's more feminine taste. Always taking tea, perhaps in the shade of another willow, the doctor, the Vicereine and later, Li's own mother would chat in private, far from the concerns of masculine China.

After having spent two years treating illiterate, lice-ridden peasants, Leonora had a lot to learn about the intricacies of Chinese etiquette. One learned to appear to eat sparingly, for example, even if ravenously hungry. Although food was constantly available and served at all hours of day and night, Leonora would always leave a little to show she had been offered more than she could eat. It was also important, when admiring Lady Li's home, not to single out a particular object, because courtesy would then require her host to make a gift of the item, and returning a gift was a terrible insult.

To give Dr. Mackenzie credit, he seems at least to have understood the glory that he would have to share with his female colleague. Leonora, having moved into the palace, was in constant attendance on the Vicereine for the next three weeks, and as she improved, word spread among the servants, officials and various hangers-on like wildfire. As Mackenzie reported: "we found that in our daily visits to our noble patient our steps were thronged with eager suppliants, who, hearing that the Viceroy's wife was undergoing medical treatment, sought for relief from the same source. You know how a story often grows as it spreads, and so this case of cure was being magnified into a miracle of healing."[6]

Miracle or not, Drs. Mackenzie and Howard would both benefit for the rest of their natural lives.

After the Vicereine had recovered, Li Hung-chang suggested that Mackenzie open a dispensary for the poor in the "Chinese City," as well as operating his clinic inside the British Concession. Mackenzie, said Li, could use the temple built in memory of Tseng Kuo-fan. Lady Li, for her own part, was bound and determined that Leonora stay in Tientsin as her personal physician, but because the lady doctor was also a missionary wishing to serve the poor, it was arranged that Leonora could operate a dispensary for women and children in the very same temple as Mackenzie. This was accomplished in October 1879.[7] It was an extremely odd arrangement, for not only were Mackenzie and Leonora members of different missionary societies, they were also doing the unheard of — treating both women and men on the same premises.

The temple was a fairly small affair, low slung and in an "L" shape, which suited the doctors' separate practices admirably. Painted red and green, the buildings were adorned with huge golden symbols assuring the late Tseng Kuo-fan prosperity in the afterlife. By Western standards it was a rude excuse for a hospital, but with money furnished by Lady Li, Leonora managed not only to dispense drugs but also to perform surgery. Within a week or so, she was treating between 30 and 50 patients a day, besides performing some serious operations, including amputations of little limbs that had become gangrenous through too-tight or dirty foot bandages. Women came from far and near for treatment, but Mary Porter of the WFMS in Peking, ever watchful of missionary interests, sent out a very earnest call for more money to build a missionary-sponsored hospital and dispensary, and also a home for Leonora in Tientsin.[8]

As a lay missionary, Miss Porter was understandably worried about the

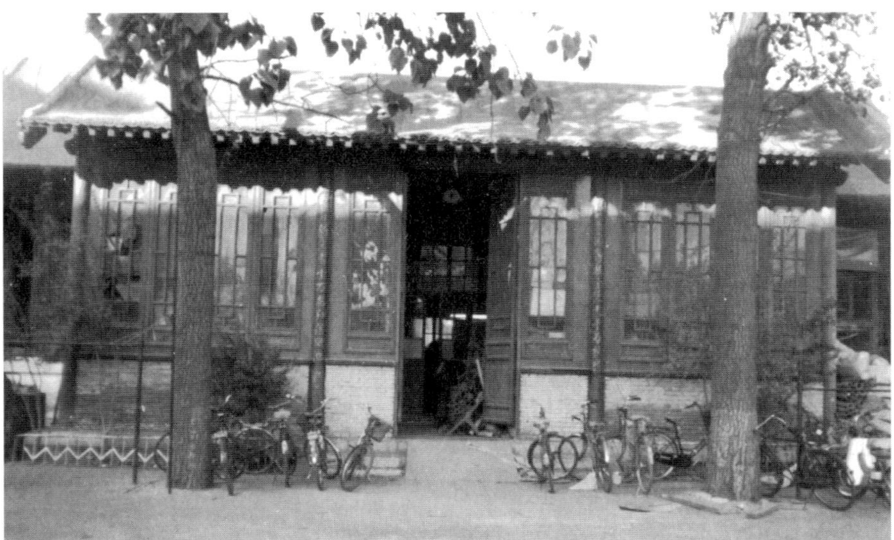

Leonora's "Temple Hospital," Tientsin

current turn of events. Addressing the WFMS assembly in 1880, she said: "It is almost impossible for Dr. Howard to give thought to the various cases presented and at the same time give religious instruction." To add to her argument, Mary Porter stressed "Dr. Howard's profession holds wide open a door that admits the multitudes to foreigners and Christians." The multitudes were indeed flocking through the door, she added, but as yet, no arrangements were being made for meeting needs "other than those of the sick, diseased bodies." In a final plea for funding, she said: "Would our Society make use of this opportunity, and grant our estimates for Tientsin, this philanthropic work would soon be established pre-eminently evangelistic."

Leonora herself seemed to be having a wonderful, if extremely busy, time at the temple. On March 21, 1880, she wrote: "The work daily becomes more interesting ... . Up to the present date I have treated 810 cases at the temple; visited 120 patients in their homes. Some of these patients resided in the city, others in the vicinity of the yamen and the temple." She had also set up a dispensary in the foreign settlement where she had taken up residence with her friends from two years ago, Reverend and Mrs. Pilcher. In her official reports, Leonora was careful to stress the importance of the settlement dispensary over the work supported by Lady Li, who was not, it seemed, a candidate for Christian conversion.

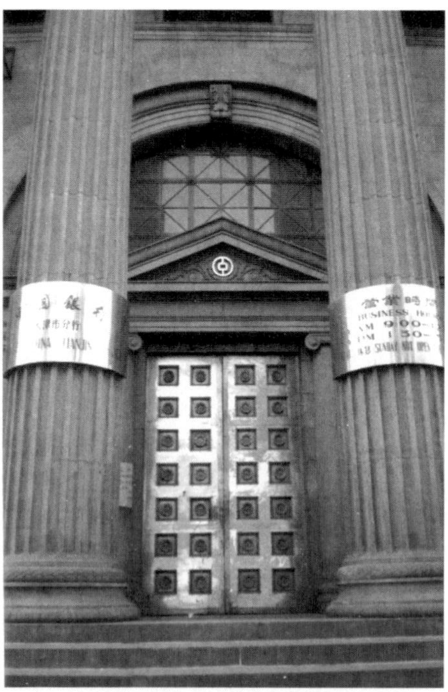

French Concession, Tientsin

"I live in the settlement," wrote the young doctor, "about three miles from the temple; have a dispensary in the settlement, and at this dispensary I have treated over 1,000 cases, and have visited 17 patients in their houses." The work in the settlement was, she stressed, entirely independent of Lady Li. Therefore, wrote Leonora winningly, "If our estimates are granted, we hope to purchase property and commence building a house and [missionary] hospital in the coming autumn." The house was in fact desperately needed, because the Pilchers had decided to build their own house, and were vacating their rental premises within the week. "Now," said Leonora, "I shall be obliged to rent a house to live in, or else give up the work in the settlement, which would not be a wise thing to do." She would also, she said, have to assume personal responsibility for renting premises that would serve as both home and dispensary.

Leonora was quickly learning that the only way to get the home boards to budge was to dangle the threat of Chinese help over Christian patronage. To sway the WFMS further, she reported: "I go to the [Lady Li's] temple every day except Sunday. I am called to the houses of the highest officials; their prejudice is breaking down everywhere over the land; patients come from the interior and take up their residence near the *temple* (author's italics), that they may be treated." The young doctor, now running her own show, fervently expressed the hope for "reinforcements" in the spring, mentioning that Mary Porter, the one whose job it was to spread the Gospel, had only managed to stay in Tientsin for two weeks in January. "While the temple work gives this work prestige," said Leonora, "this work is of more importance from a missionary standpoint. You can see" she wrote firmly, "how the matter stands."[9]

Endnotes

1. Latourette, Kenneth. *A History of Christian Missions in China*. London: Society for Promoting Christian Knowledge, 1929, p. 454.
2. Dr. Irwin, though mentioned briefly in a missionary list, seems to have disappeared off the face of the map. The author can find no further reference to him.
3. Li's secretary for more than 25 years was an American named Pethick.
4. Hodgkins, Louise Manning. *The Roll Call*. Boston: Woman's Foreign Missionary Society, 1896, p. 15.
5. Although Mackenzie asserts that Leonora spent a month in the palace, the Woman's Foreign Missionary Society reports she was in residence for three weeks.
6. *Chinese Recorder* 22, p. 478.
7. *Eleventh Annual Report of the Woman's Foreign Missionary Society*. Chicago: 1880, pp. 33-34.
8. Ibid., pp. 33-34.
9. Ibid., pp. 33-34.

Chapter twelve

The women
1880

Here am I: for thou calledst me.
— I Samuel 5:5

Leonora began to build a small but effective, all-female missionary empire. In answer to her "earnest call for help,"[1] the WFMS had sent out two more American ladies. There were now five full-time workers, all single women: Leonora, Clara Cushman, Mary Porter, and the newcomers Annie B. Sears from the Cincinnati branch and Elizabeth Yates from the New England branch. Two wives, Mrs. Lowry and Mrs. Davis, worked alongside.

"To meet the great demand created by Dr. Howard's success during her short visit to Tientsin," wrote the Home Board, "the appointment of the ladies to their work was left to the missionary authorities in N. China, and it seems from Miss Porter's report that very satisfactory arrangements have been made." The new missionaries, Misses Sears and Yates, stayed in Peking with Mary Porter, learning the language and helping with the schoolchildren. Clara Cushman, a bit more seasoned in the field, joined Leonora in Tientsin until the school year ended, when she changed places with Mary Porter.

Mary was eager to establish a missionary "training school" in Tientsin, but felt she should remain in Peking while school was in session. "We all agree that this arrangement meets all requirements," wrote Mary Porter. "Tientsin needs some one who can talk, that will leave a big burden on some one in Pekin [sic]. I have been here longest and therefore can meet needs of Pekin [sic] alone, better than another more recently out." Mary had, she noted, one of the most advanced classes, and could "carry them on easily and have girls help me with Miss Cushman's classes ... Miss Cushman will have time to study and get ready to take my classes, and by that time new ladies will be able to help considerable [sic]."

As noted previously, Mary Porter was determined that the word of God should enter Leonora's Chinese-donated temple as quickly as possible. The Misses Sears or Yates in Tientsin, she wrote, could do nothing but study, and the "talking" at the temple dispensary would not be done. Setting up a missionary training school for her Chinese Bible Women would have to be delayed, owing to the perennial problem of housing. "If Miss Cushman is in Tientsin to teach and talk to Dr. Howard's patients the evangelistic work among women of Tientsin will have a beginning and the training school can wait, indeed it will have to wait, as the houses are not yet built." Mary proposed to spend several weeks at a time in various country stations, teaching the women and getting acquainted, "Thus I shall be able to judge who is best fitted to taking into the city for further instructions."

Like Leonora and many missionaries to come, Mary found it easier to work with uneducated, rural women, many of whom were more quickly swayed from their rude lives of domestic slavery. "I am more and more satisfied that there is a great and most promising field of labor in these country districts among the simple-hearted, cordial, village women," she wrote. But like every missionary who had spent at least a year in China, she had to be honest with herself about the prospects of conversion. "No doubt vague hopes of pecuniary gain hauuts [haunts] the hearts of some of the poor creatures and adds warmth to their welcome to the foreigner whose resources seem unlimited ... but when they learn that sacrifice and devotion is asked for Christ's sake and no money paid the true will come to the front ... ." Determined to set the Home Board's minds at ease, she quickly added, "there are true ones no doubt."

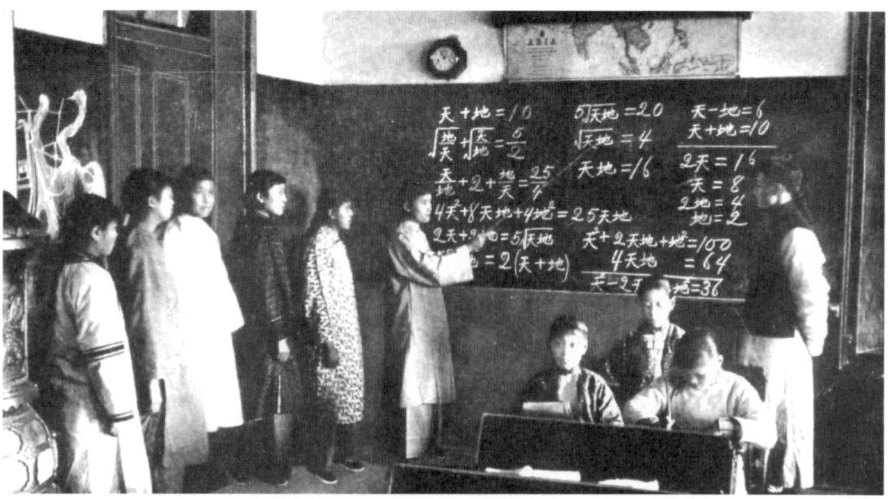

Algebra class, Chinkiang Girls' School

The missionary training school meant a great deal of country work, with at least six months' teaching "of women collected from Christian homes in various villages and brought to the city, then send women back ... to teach and preach ... then make a long visit to each place, encouraging, inspiring, teaching, and meeting with people. Then another six months in school and visits again and so on through each year." Conversion work was arduous and to some missionaries it seemed pointless to go on. Mary Porter, who like Leonora would remain in China for most of her life, was cautious, reporting, "During a revival of a few weeks, several of our girls were received on probation. I note a change in the conduct of several that indicates a change of purpose, and I trust," she added tartly, "a change of heart."

Leonora herself, worked to the bone, now fell sick with the first of many bouts of malaria. This debilitating illness was common in Tientsin, because the city was surrounded by swampland — ideal territory for the mosquitoes that carried the dread infection. Malaria reputedly refers to *mal aria*,[2] meaning "evil air," and during the summer months the air in Tientsin was evil indeed. Leonora suffered through alternate chills and fever, anemia, and an enlarged spleen. Weakened by vomiting and diarrhea, she may have lapsed into delirium or even coma.

Luckily an effective treatment was known long before the cause of this disease was understood. Western legend had it that Jesuits learned about the bark of a certain tree in Peru as far back as 1630. From 1700 onward this bark's most active ingredient, quinine, became the universal treatment for malaria. The importance of quinine cannot be overstated, for without it many of the fertile lands in the world would not have been habitable. But quinine's chief shortcoming was that it could not eradicate any relapsing infections. From this early bout with Tientsin's scourge, general poor health would plague Leonora for the rest of her life.

Owing to her illness, she had not sent a report back to the WFMS since October 6, 1880. She then wrote: "I am much stronger than was the case one month ago, and shall be satisfied to do the best I can alone, if you can only get a physician for Pekin [sic]." Travelling back and forth was becoming too much for any one person to bear, let alone someone suffering from the after-effects of malaria. Hundreds of patients poured in from the countryside. For the last quarter Leonora reported 670 new patients at the temple and "1,621 old patients; total, 2,291. Patients in the foreign settlement hospital* have numbered 750; outside patients [those whose homes she visited], 63."

*This was not a hospital, but a dispensary operated from Leonora's home.

In her own report to the Home Board, missionary Clara Cushman offered her support, saying bluntly that "The above figures are a sufficient explanation for no later reports from Dr. Howard's overtaxed hands." But the women still shared some humour about their hard work. On January 27, 1881, Clara offered a rather amusing description of the women's joint efforts. "Dr. Howard has one woman under treatment from whose head she removed a tumor of 30 years' growth," she wrote. "The head is doing well and I am trying to lead the poor heart to Jesus."[3]

But 30 year-old tumours aside, Leonora was faced with many more appalling cases, some brought on through the Chinese "customs" of footbinding and wife and daughter-in-law abuse, others through a combination of superstition and lack of sanitation. Add to this a want of proper nourishment, shelter and heat, the myriads of germ-laden mosquitoes and the unhindered multiplication of fleas, flies, bedbugs and lice, and it was no wonder practically everyone had something wrong with them. Fellow Canadian Dr. James Frazer Smith would later write that after careful observation, a fair estimate indicated that "seven out of every ten persons in the average crowd ... were in need of medical treatment or surgical aid." Many of the cases were critical, and others hopeless.

Leonora must have marvelled at the resilience of the Chinese to a number of diseases such as blood poisoning, dysentery, typhoid and smallpox, but there was little stamina in cases of pneumonia, malarial fever, and plague. The theory of "survival of the fittest" certainly rang true in 19th-century China. It is interesting to note that since foreigners fell like flies when exposed to disease, Leonora, exposed to every germ imaginable, must have been in robust health to have lived through her own bout with malaria.

The women and their children came from miles around, lice infested and filthy, and with suppurating sores and scabs. While the lay missionaries were aware of the poverty, misery and wretchedness of the common people, the gentle Leonora, needing to question patients about wounds and infections, came to know the most intimate details of their lives. Working 12 hours a day, sometimes more, she had little more than her medical bag, some fairly crude medicines, and a small temple with a dirt floor.

Leonora's medical kit consisted of scalpels, some fine enough to remove cataracts, a magnifying glass for close work, and forceps for extracting teeth. At her back-door clinic, at her temple "hospital" and everywhere on field trips, both men and women would gather, with their pus-laden boils, nasty red felons,* painful abscesses, and plain old toothache. At times more than a dozen

*A felon is an inflammatory sore on the finger, near the nail.

might silently line up, pointing to their jaws and mimicking agony. Nearly every medical missionary has written with amazement at the stoic attitude of the Chinese, who never made a sound during surgery, even work done without anaesthetic. When peoples' offending molars were removed, wrote one doctor, the Chinese would simply walk away with great happy smiles.[4]

Then there was the physical slavery of women — the extraordinarily cruel custom of binding a young child's feet. Han Chinese women — the ruling Manchus did not bind their feet — were in absolute fact crippled to prevent them from running away, and could not walk without the help of sticks or servants upon whom to lean. More appalling was the fact that mothers who had themselves experienced this agony were required by society to inflict the pain on their own daughters. A girl with big feet was not marriageable.

In May 1870, Dr. John Dudgeon of the London Missionary Society in Peking dwelt on the medical effects of bound feet. "The decreased physical activity ... often caused ... slowed-down circulation, loss of appetite and menstrual disorders that might prevent conception," he said. And Lin Shou-pao, a progressive Chinese Baptist at Cheffoo noted, against everything believed by his countrymen, that footbinding was an "artificial" way of enhancing female attractiveness and that women were prevented from realizing their full potential. Furthermore, he said, since a large number of women, disabled by footbinding, played no part in economic life, the country's production was affected, resulting in "the poverty of the state and people."[5] Christianity was beginning to work in mysterious political ways.

Then there was the common custom of beating women. One teenager came to Leonora's Tientsin hospital with "a terrible eye." She was accompanied by an older woman who did all the talking. "Her name is Mu," said the older woman. "She is twenty-three years old. She has a small child six months old, a girl. When it was born the whole family were angry because it was a girl, and they beat her. Her mother-in-law has beaten her ever since. She beat her on her eye and made it like that." Another, with her face all swollen and bruised, pointed at her own little child and said: "Her father beat me." Another old patient standing by spoke up: "Yes, all Chinese beat their wives. Here I am seventy years old, and my hair is gray and still I have to be beaten."

It is only fair to note here that although wife-beating was not limited to the lower classes, the richer Chinese men tended to leave that unsavoury duty to their own mothers. It was a system of calculated vengeance — if it had happened to them, they in turn would inflict it upon someone else. In wealthier households the beatings generally stopped when a son and heir was produced.

But the daughters of slaves, the daughters of servants, and the daughters of peasants continued to be scalded with boiling water or oil, starved, and pinched until their bruises actually burst. One day two young girls, one well-dressed and strong, the other thin, sick, hollow-eyed and clothed in rags, came into Leonora's waiting room. "This is my sister," began the older one, "and she has a mother-in-law who hates her. She is fourteen years old ... just look at her hands," she said, pointing to hard, blackened little hands that looked as if they had scrubbed and cleaned continually. "She has to work all the time and they wont [sic] give her any good clothes and they beat her!" the sister said, growing more excited every minute. "They not only treat her in that manner but, doctor, they *won't give her food*."

The reason for this maltreatment was that the young girl's husband had given her a "bad sickness" — most probably syphilis — and "they all hate her because she has it, and want her to die." When the foreign lady doctor asked, "But why don't your father and mother help her?" the older girl said, "Why, we don't know anything about them! We were both sold when we were little ones."

But hope shone on the horizon for the beaten and starved women of Chihli Province. The missionaries' desperate pleas for funding had been answered by a Methodist philanthropist in Baltimore. Leonora watched her own modern hospital being built, day after glorious day.

Endnotes

1. *Twelfth Annual Report of the Woman's Foreign Missionary Society*. Chicago: The Society, 1881, p. 34.
2. "Malaria: History," *Encyclopedia Britannica* 14. London: Encyclopedia Britannica Inc., 1967, p. 669.
3. *Twelfth Annual Report of the Woman's Foreign Missionary Society*. Chicago: The Society, 1880-81, p. 34.
4. Frazer Smith, Reverend James, MD, CM. *Life's Waking Part*. Toronto: Thomas Nelson & Sons, 1937, p. 104.
5. Fairbank, John K. *The Missionary Enterprise in China and America*. Cambridge, Mass.: Harvard University Press, 1974, p. 187.

Chapter thirteen

Alex arrives
1880–1886

Behold, I stand at the door, and knock.
— Revelation 3:20

The Isabella Fisher Hospital for Women and Children was named for a sister of Mrs. John Goucher of Baltimore. Responding to the urgent appeals from Peking and Tientsin, Mrs. Goucher and her husband had donated $5,000 to Leonora's cause. It was, in fact, much easier to obtain funds than to start on the building process itself. Because the hospital was to be built in the "Chinese City" rather than the foreign settlement, land purchase had become a major problem, owing to the Chinese manner of protracted business dealings and the ever-present system of graft. In February 1881, Mary Porter wrote that "The only land to be had for Tientsin work has been purchased at great expense after long delay. Obstacles and hindrances that could not be foreseen have made it necessary to almost double the amount we expected to pay for land and walls, and now we are obliged to ask for more ... the hospital buildings and [Leonora's] house may now be under way. The land has to be filled and walled in and will cost when done more than was anticipated ... ."[1]

Soon enough an additional amount of $2,000 was supplied by the generous Gouchers of Baltimore. How delighted Leonora must have been to finally realize her dream of clean, modern facilities and her very own home. She may, in fact, have been the first spinster missionary in China who did not have to share premises with a married couple. Independence and autonomy undreamed of in North America had been granted through the curious combination of one royal Chinese woman and a middle-class couple in the United States.

The *Chinese Recorder* proudly reported that the Isabella Fisher Hospital:

> "under the care of Miss Dr. Howard of the American Methodist Episcopal Mission, was formally opened for the

> reception and treatment of women and children, by the Reverend Bishop Bowman on October 15th [1881]. A goodly number of foreign friends were present, together with a large representation from the four native churches. The exercises were partly in Chinese and partly in English. The Scripture read was taken from Matthew 9, xviii-xxxviii. Prayer was then offered, after which the hymn "The Great Physician" was sung, followed by a brief statement of the origin of the medical mission work for women in Peking, and the circumstances which lead [sic] to the erection of this hospital in particular. After this, Bishop Bowman gave an address, and dedicated the institution by prayer to the uses for which it had been erected. At the close of the dedicatory exercises, the friends were invited to inspect the premises.
>
> "They [the premises] are situated on the great road leading from Tientsin to Taku, a few rods West of the English concession. The main building has a hall running through from front to rear, and contains a large waiting room and two smaller private rooms, a well-supplied dispensing room, a fine drug room and an admirably lighted operating room. Back of this main building are wards on three sides of a court, so situated as to get the benefit of the sun's heat and light to the best advantage. One of these, the general ward, is arranged to accommodate 24 patients. The other buildings contain four rooms each, and will accommodate 16 patients, or by crowding, twice that number could be placed in them temporarily. The place is well-situated, well-ventilated, and amply furnished with kitchens and other necessary outbuildings. Including the purchase of the land, and the enclosing wall, the hospital has cost about $6,000."

Now bereft of Leonora's services in Peking, Mary Porter again began lobbying for more staff. In her inimitable fashion of stating a strong but carefully polite case, she wrote: "You cannot imagine what variety a missionary lady has in her work. From building a house to making beef tea for the sick; making books and teaching housekeeping and itinerating; all the family cares of a mother with 36 girls to clothe, feed and do her own teaching; preaching and teaching, superintending girls at washing; searching bodies of those suspected of being untidy [many children had lice]; reports, day schools, Sunday-school lessons and all extra moments to scholarship letters. You can see," she said rather plaintively, "that we need the inspiration of a letter to answer when we snatch a few moments to write to the interested supporters of our girls. We long for the coming of medical ladies to Pekin [sic]. This Chinese city work would move off nicely with a dispensary to draw in the people in our new quarters."

In the meantime Leonora seemed destined to rise to fame, both in China and abroad. Reverend Pilcher, with whose family Leonora had been boarding, praised her unremitting work to the Parent Board. "To me it seems impossible to overestimate the work already done. It cannot be that nearly five thousand women, many of whom have been saved from imminent death, should go away without a new conception of life and a thought of the Gospel which gives birth to such benevolence and such sacrifice."

Then, through another short paragraph in Pilcher's report, Leonora gained a different type of fame. "Another significant providence in Dr. Howard's work for Christ is seen," wrote Pilcher, "in the facts connected with the very favorable treaty the United States has recently secured with China, through the new American Minister at the court of Pekin [sic], Dr. Angell, formerly president of the University of Michigan." Pilcher, in his enthusiasm to impress the Home Board, would now drop a bombshell that would reverberate all the way to Washington, DC. "Dr. Howard graduated at Michigan University," he wrote, "and President Angell's name was upon her diploma. Hence when Lady Li asked Dr. Howard if Mr. Angell was a good man, her answer can be readily conceived. Lady Li responded, 'If you say he is good he must be good.' "

This incident, reported Reverend Pilcher, "had its influence in disposing Viceroy Li to listen with confidence and kindness to the words of President Angell, and so the Gospel of the Prince of peace promotes peace and thus is fulfilled the prophecy of Isaiah. 'Violence shall no more be heard in thy land; wasting nor destruction within thy borders; but thou shalt call thy word's salvation and thy gates praise.' "

Considering Leonora's quiet dedication and reluctance to write detailed reports, it is difficult to understand how this piece of news came about. It is highly unlikely that Leonora herself went around trumpeting the *coup*, and we cannot, therefore, be entirely sure of its accuracy. To their dying days, neither Li Hung-chang nor his wife spoke any English, preferring to communicate through Li's secretary Pethick, who would hardly have made such a diplomatic blunder as to broadcast this news. Leonora did speak Chinese by this time, but that in itself would have no bearing on the case. In such a patriarchal society, it is difficult to entertain the notion that Lady Li had much influence over her husband's political decisions, particularly regarding crucial foreign treaties. To give both Li and his wife the benefit of the doubt, Li was in almost constant contact with powerful Empress Dowager, Tz'u-hsi, and having experience with women and politics, he may, as many politicians before and afterward, have privately consulted with his wife.

It would be interesting to think that Leonora did have some influence here. Perhaps she did meet Dr. Angell while he was ambassador, but because of the heavy line drawn between diplomat and missionary, she would only have done so through her contacts with the Viceroy's family. Knowing that Li was dealing with Angell, she may very well have mentioned to Lady Li that the latter had been president of her university in the United States, and this could have led to something resembling influence. Angell himself, when pushed by a number of people for some sort of explanation, remained silent.

The treaty in question limited Chinese immigration to the United States, and included an "opium clause" prohibiting Americans from trading in the odious drug. Chinese immigration was beginning to be felt, not only in coastal areas such as California but also farther inland on the railroads and eventually in such places as New York. As immigrants they were distinctly unwelcome. Just before Angell left for China, Reverend O. Gibson wrote to him, saying: "While I do not share in the woful [sic] prophecies of impending ruin to our country on account of Chinese immigration, still, I am ready to admit there are certain objections to a large Chinese immigration, which do not exist in the case of any other people who come in any considerable numbers to our shores. Their dissimilarity in dress and general social customs, and their slowness to assimilate to the forms and customs of our civilization, lie at the base of all the real objections to the presence of this people among us, and present a constant occasion for race prejudice and friction.

"Certainly," wrote Gibson, "no statesman will seriously object to this immigration on account of its industry and economy. But while our institutions propose a government of the people by the people, we still open wide our door to free immigration from all lands. We do this however with the underlying idea and expectation that all the peoples who immigrate to our country, come with the intent and purpose of making this country their permanent home, the native country of their children. We expect that immigration ... will rapidly become thoroughly American in idea, purpose and loyalty to our government and institution.

"It has occurred to me that if there should be presented to the Chinese government, a calm and fair statement of this fundamental cause of friction ... that government might be induced to issue a proclamation in China, permitting its subjects who wish to immigrate to America to lay aside the queue and Chinese dress, and adopt the American costume without forfeiting the protection of the Chinese government."

There now emerged a distinct prejudice in the reverend's suggestions, because he followed with this. "The knowledge of the fact that all Chinese immigrating to America would be required to cut off the queue, and adopt American social customs, would lessen the rate of immigration more than fifty per cent."

Reverend Gibson did have some understanding of what he called the Chinese "custom" of wearing the queue, but he didn't quite seem to understand that cutting it off was absolute treason, punishable by death, in Manchu-ruled China. He noted that "it is a badge of loyalty to the reigning dynasty," but blithely added that "it is this and it is nothing more." His proposed action, he asserted, "would relieve the Chinese in America from much embarrassment, race prejudice and wicked persecution," and "tend to limit the immigration and vastly improve all that came." Now Gibson's true colours began to emerge. "So long as he nurses this badge of allegiance to the Chinese government the Chinaman will make but slow progress in adopting the higher forms of our Christian civilization."

An obvious question emerges concerning Westerners in China, such as Leonora herself, who chose to remain clothed in occidental fashion. But Gibson, in his own prejudice, had an answer for everything. "The astute Chinese diplomat will doubtless meet this ... with the counter proposition that all Americans in China shall conform to Chinese dress and social customs. But the cases are not parallel. The American residents in China are comparatively few in number, and are composed for the most part of our well-educated and enterprising citizens, professional and commercial men. So that the disparity in dress and habits of life does not create that friction with the masses of China, which is created in America by the tons of uneducated and unskilled Chinese ... who come here to compete in our labor market, with the uneducated and unskilled working classes from all other parts of the world."

It is fairly obvious that Gibson, living in the United States, had never been stared at, poked, pulled, pushed and threatened by Chinese villagers who shouted "Foreign Devil!" when Westerners, clothed as such, entered their various enclaves. It is equally obvious that he had never had mud slung at him, rocks pelted at him, or been threatened with decapitation simply because he looked different from the Chinese. But in this parallel, at least, his carefully worded letter to Angell had a point: it is a fact of most, if not all, societies that alien dress, accents and mannerisms leave a person wide open to criticism, persecution, and sometimes violence. Chinese workers in both Canada and the United States were, in fact, treated abominably by most white people.

By November 1880, James Angell had successfully concluded the terms of his Sino-American treaty, with Li Hung-chang acting on behalf of the

Emperor. News of Leonora's supposed influence began to appear in the newspapers. According to the Peking correspondent of the *New York Herald*, who must have been talking to Mr. Pilcher, much of the credit for this treaty should have been given to Dr. Leonora Howard. The news of her supposed coup flashed across the United States and letters began pouring into Peking. Angell's friend Rowland Hazard wrote an enthusiastic letter November 28, stating:

> "we are much excited [about] the statement which appears to be authorized that you have concluded a satisfactory treaty in this Commission and are returning with it. This is great news almost too good to be true — If it is true I shall see in it the hand of the Lord working in a way that sets at nought mans [sic] wisdom. Who could forsee [sic] that when Miss Howard entered your College, where in the course of the discharge of your duty, she learned to respect you not only as an officer of the College but as a Christian gentleman — When you signed your name to her diploma I say who could forsee that when these steps were taken you were fitting the Key which was to open the doors of Chinese diplomacy.
>
> Yet luck seems to have been the result — Miss Howard obtained by her skill the entrie into Prince Li Chungs [sic] family. Miss Howard when asked by Madame Li about you could reply in terms of admiring esteem. This confidence of Li Chung [sic] was thus won & the whole matter became simple. This is the way I read the riddle—I do not think I can be far wrong. The beautiful thing about this is that the steps you took were the simple steps of duty seen at the time, and you knew not whither they would land. Truly blessed is it to feel that if we walk in the path of duty our Father will see to it that the path leads us whithersoever he would have us go.

Other colleagues expressed more scepticism. On December 6, an associate named Hannah wrote that "The report of the interview between Li H.C. and the woman who graduated at A.A. had ... concerning you at first [amused?] us and if true is certainly a remarkable coincidence. The [undecipherable] the correspondent of the *N.Y. Herald* made a tremendous long matter of it in his last letter."

The most hostile comments came from Angell's own son, Alexander, or "Eck." It took Eck until May 1881 to write to his father about the rumours. A rather bitter outpouring reads as follows: "A letter has been going the rounds of the papers from your accurate Chinese correspondent of the *N.Y. Herald* in which it is said that Miss Howard the physician moved Lady Li to move Lord

Li to move the Yaman [sic] to move the Emperor to make your treaty, that it was due to Miss H.'s representation that you were a 'good man' that you had any success at all. If this can be shown by affidavit after the ratification Miss H. should have the worst looking old blue glass brass mounted Heathen Curio to be found in Yannan."[2]

Eck's defence of his father, if overly heated, is perfectly understandable, given the times. Women physicians were frowned upon, and anything that would take credit away from Ambassador Angell would inevitably reflect upon his son's own place in society. Suffice it to say that there remained two schools of thought about Leonora's involvement.

In 1882, the call for another woman physician was answered in the form of Dr. L.E. Akers. Like Leonora, she spent most of her first year of service in language training. Other medical women were now moving slowly into central, southern and Western China, and their work began to be well-recognized at home. The *Chinese Recorder* noted:

> "The importance of the work done by Lady Physicians ... in Canton where foreign medical missionary work has been carried on for many years, there has been some change in sentiment on the part of the people, and it is reported that a third of the patients at the missionary hospital have been women ... . it is true that Chinese women are beyond the reach of the male physicians ... we must express the hope that this branch of missionary work in China will be more frequently and more fully reported than it has been in the past."[3]

Elizabeth Yates was quick to point out the lay missionaries' own involvement with Leonora's hospitals, writing: "My heart knows something of the 'hundred fold' of joy promised to those who leave home and friends for Christ, when from the lips of these heathen children I hear —

> 'Jesus the water of life will give,
> Freely, freely, freely,'

and the ear of faith hears the mighty chorus that shall one day arise from this nation ... ." Miss Yates, like many other new arrivals, truly believed that China's millions would one day be united in Christianity.

That winter Elizabeth Yates acted mostly as a translator for fellow newcomer Dr. Akers, allowing Leonora to continue her work both in town and out. "Since the weather became warmer," she wrote, "I have been engaged in teaching twenty-three in-patients [at the Isabella Fisher Hospital]." The WFMS women had also recruited a Bible Woman, Mrs. Wang, who took over proselytizing at the gates of Leonora's home-cum-dispensary. "When the weather is suitable patients come daily to the Dispensary," reported Dr. Akers. "Mrs. Wang ... scatters the precious seed among the patients, as my other duties take all my time. During all the year I have held Monday afternoon meetings for women in my study, with an attendance varying from five to twenty-five."

It is interesting to note that this early, at least one woman missionary was allowed to preach in church. "Since the 4th of July," Miss Yates wrote, "I have had them in the Chapel, which has opened new work to me. I intended to have a service once a week, but the interest seemed to warrant their daily continuance." Attendance during the week totalled 70 Chinese, "among whom were more than a dozen men, some of whom apparently were of the literati, who listened with respectful attention." This was, she wrote, "the first service of the kind ever undertaken by a lady. It has the support and sympathy of the gentlemen of our mission."

Leonora herself reported that the work sponsored by Lady Li was, for the time being, on hold. And Lady Li was ill once more. "The Temple Dispensary has not been opened during the past year," she wrote. "First, because of my purpose last fall to go home;[4] second, the premises for some months have been occupied by a Viceroy and his retinue. Excepting twelve weeks of the winter months our Mission Dispensary has been opened daily, seven weeks of which I spent in constant medical attendance on Lady Li, the remainder of the time on a country trip, in company with Miss Cushman."

During this time, Leonora said, Dr. Akers opened the Isabella Fisher dispensary twice a week, and visited outpatients when sent for. "I kept no statistics of work done by me while in the country," she said. "A goodly number came to the Mission premises, eager to get medicine. While I tried to relieve physical suffering, Miss Cushman told them of the great Physician. Some too ill to come out invited us to visit them in their homes." This was probably a "first" in any field trip made by any China missionary. "In every instance," wrote Leonora, "we were treated with confidence and respect."

Leonora was obviously pleased with the way things were going, and wrote highly of her colleagues. "Miss Yates," she said, "has held daily service in the Hospital wards, doing faithful and effective work in spreading God's truth." [Bible Woman] "Miss [sic] Wang has been very helpful and trustworthy, never losing an opportunity to speak for the Master." Dr. Howard also had good words for her male associates. "Since the establishment of my work in city or country, I have been indebted to the gentlemen of the mission for kindness, counsel and hearty co-operation."[5]

One of these gentlemen was Reverend Alexander King, born March 5, 1850, at Kintore, Aberdeenshire, Scotland. A tall, quiet, lanky young man, he seemed to have lost his parents at an early age. Members of Scotland's lower middle class lived in genteel poverty, with a joint of mutton or perhaps a precious lamb chop served but rarely. Church was central to the lives of these conservative people, and each Sunday parishioners like Alex and his one sister gave what little money they had, rather than exchange their worn but still-serviceable clothes for newer, more fashionable garb.

There is no record about Alex's decision to enter the ministry and then to embark on a missionary career, but it is likely that he, like many others, saw ahead of him nothing but a dreary life of repairing leaky church roofs, visiting the sick in the cold Scottish drizzle, and presiding at stuffy church teas. Surely, thought many young people, there was more to religion than that. In any event, Alex decided that a churchman's life overseas was appropriate to his beliefs and perhaps to his carefully suppressed *joie de vivre*, which would later charm people everywhere, from Chinese converts to Leonora's own family.

Alex King embarked upon his dreams rather late, graduating from Spring Hill College at age 30. On January 8, 1880, he married Elizabeth Wilson in the Church of Scotland at Aberdeen. Six days later Alex was ordained at Carr's Lane Church, Birmingham (Dale), and, on January 30, the novice missionaries set sail for China.[6]

Elizabeth, like more than half the women who went into the field as wives, was married just days before her departure. We don't know if she chose Alex for love alone, or whether her marriage combined a religious commitment with a romantic one. Although many wives entered the field because they had married ordained ministers, sometimes the decision was made by the woman herself. Pearl Buck, famous for her many books about China, reported that her mother, Carrie Sydenstricker, had resolved to become a missionary at her mother's deathbed, and married for her soul, rather than her heart. Another well-known missionary, Jeanie Graham, had broken off several romances because the suitors did not share her commitment to missionary service.[7]

Alex and Elizabeth stayed in Hong Kong for two days, then spent four days in Shanghai before setting off for Tientsin, their final destination. Little did they know how very final it would be. On April 16, 1880, Alex wrote, "I was surprised and glad to find such a thriving mission organized in Tientsin, for although the converts are very, very few ... still ... I was delighted to see the daily morning prayer and church meeting so well attended." The newly married Kings stayed with another London missionary, Jonathan Lees, and Alex wrote with hope that "arrangements have been made for accommodations till a house shall have been provided for us which I trust will be done without delay." Like others before him, he was in for a long wait.

On August 5, Jonathan Lees wrote to the Home Board in London. "As to Mr. King's house, on his arrival we were already far advanced with our new hospital scheme, but temporarily stopped for want of [dollars]. The Directors' inability to help us, though disappointing, was not unexpected ... no premises at all suitable could be had under from taels 300 to taels 400 per annum ... it occurred to me that the right thing to do would be to build another of the hospital wards already planned and to fit it up with temporary partitions ... in such a way that it might serve our brother's purpose as a dwelling house for a short time ... ."

Alex and Elizabeth's daughter was born October 7, 1880, exactly 10 months after their marriage. Although he must have been overjoyed, the careful Scot was determined to exercise his fiscal responsibility. On November 20, Alex sent his report to London. "I write to inform you that a child — a daughter was born to us the 7th of October and to ask that the usual allowance be made for her." Regarding his new fieldwork, he had as yet little to say, noting: "I am of course principally occupied in acquiring the language — and difficult and tedious work I find it ... at present I can read the language better than I can speak it. But now that I have got hold of a good many simple phrases, I shall, I hope soon be able ... to understand their speech and be understood by them. ... I long to be able to talk to the people, for here there is no difficulty in getting crowds of listeners."

Tragically, Elizabeth Wilson King died March 3, 1881, due to heart and lung complications brought on by typhoid fever. Although Drs. Mackenzie and Irwin were in residence with the London Missionary Society, she may well have been tended by Leonora Howard. But nothing could be done about the virulence of her fever, and Elizabeth succumbed in just 10 days.

"We regret to hear of the death of Mrs. King, wife of the Reverend Alexander King, of the London Missionary Society," wrote the Reverend C.A. Stanley. "Mrs. King reached Tientsin with her husband less than a year ago, but during these few months [she] had won the love and esteem of all who knew her. She was a woman of much character and promise. She leaves a babe of about five months. ... she suffered much during the progress of the disease, but her end was peaceful and happy."[8]

New husband, new father, and novice missionary, Alex must have reeled in shock at this turn of events. But he was not unique in his grief. Prior to the missionary societies' establishment of "resort" areas where the air and water were cleaner, new arrivals died with alarming regularity, most commonly of malaria, diphtheria, cholera, and dysentery. Carrie Sydenstricker lost four of her seven children, then blamed herself, as if it were her own sins that killed her little ones. Other missionaries wrote that maybe God felt they were not concentrating enough on their missionary work, and that they were being punished.[9]

But tragedy refused to leave the unhappy Minister. Alex's baby daughter, whose name is unknown, died of smallpox on May 13, just weeks after her mother's own death. Alex, shattered, had once more to put pen to paper. "Dear Sir," he wrote to London, "I write to thank you for your kind letter of sympathy with reference to the death of my dear wife: and I have now to inform you that the very day I received your letter my only child died of smallpox." Bereft of everything dear to him, Alex turned to the Lord. "I trust that despite these trials I may still be enabled to carry on my work here with unabated trust in God."[10]

The missionary community was still small, and social occasions few and far between, but somehow love was allowed to flourish. Three years later, on August 21, 1884, the Reverend H.H. Lowrie joined Dr. Leonora Annetta Howard and the Reverend Alexander King in holy matrimony. Leonora changed her name to Dr. *Ke ye-da*, the Chinese version of King.* The next day, August 22, the French declared war on China.

Endnotes

1. *Twelfth Annual Report of the Woman's Foreign Missionary Society*. Chicago: The Society, 1881, pp. 35-39.
2. Michigan Historical Collections, Bentley Historical Library, University of Michigan. Various Commissions and Diplomatic Missions. Box 2, China Section, No. 13. Alexander (Eck) Angell to his father, May 1881.
3. *Chinese Recorder* 15, p. 23.
4. Leonora did not actually return home that year.
5. *Fourteenth Annual Report of the Woman's Foreign Missionary Society*. Chicago: The Society, 1883, pp. 29-30.
6. Register of L.M.S. Missionaries. London: School of Oriental and African Studies, University of London, p. 104.
7. Hunter, Jane. *The Gospel of Gentility - American Women Missionaries in Turn-of-the-Century China*. New Haven: Yale University Press, 1984, p. 90.
8. *Chinese Recorder* 12, pp. 134, 139.
9. Hunter, Jane. *The Gospel of Gentility*, pp. 119-120.
10. Council for World Missionary Archives, Day Missions Library, Yale University. London Missionary Society Records. Box 4-1881, No. 83. June 20, 1881.

*It is not known what Leonora's Chinese name was before this. It could have been something like Hu-wa. Dr. Mackenzie is known to this day as "Dr. Ma."

Chapter fourteen

The Canadians
1885

Be not righteous over much.
— Ecclesiastes 7:16

Leonora's marriage to Alex King had necessitated resigning from the WFMS. Even though the General Boards were, for the times, remarkably lenient with women in the field, they all agreed that a woman's place was alongside her husband. If the husband, like Alex, happened to belong to another missionary society, Leonora's sad lot would be to leave her cherished Isabella Fisher Hospital and assist her husband in his own work of preaching the Gospel for the British. But surprisingly this was not to be the case, and the London Missionary Society (LMS) did not seem to realize that she kept going her own way. Although Alex King belonged to the LMS, Leonora never did work in an official capacity for that organization, because Lady Li had now decided to build her a brand-new hospital of her very own. This rather startling development naturally had an effect on Alex's own work, and his immediate supervisor, Jonathan Lees, wrote that with regard to a new mission planned for the interior, "Mr. King ... indeed since his marriage, seems wavering on the subject in a manner which is to me personally a little discouraging."[1]

Lees had a right to be discouraged, for after five years in China, Alex was turning into an asset, rather than as had first been felt, a bit of a liability. At this point, the lanky churchman still had trouble with the language, but with Leonora's help he was on his way to becoming fluent. Alex had, like a number of other male missionaries, quite a bit of trouble learning Chinese, and indeed had written about his difficulty to the Home Board. As the Reverend Lees suggested, perhaps Alex's age (though 35 was not exactly old) had something to do with it.[2] In any case, women did seem to have a better ability to pick up the tones and various nuances the language. But by the time he married Leonora, Alex seemed to be making good progress in reading and writing Chinese. As a churchman, he recognized that it was all-important to master verbal communication.

Now that Alex had a reasonable, if not perfect command of the language, combined with the tremendous asset of a medical wife, the LMS began to look at him as a bit more of an asset. His gentleness and goodness seemed to match Leonora's, and they both genuinely liked the Chinese. Alex was reported to be "Very unobtrusive, much at home in work amongst the villages, and with a deep fund of kindliness (of which advantage was sometimes taken), he won a very secure place in the affections of the Chinese."[3] This was not necessarily true of other missionaries, who were alternately disgusted, afraid of, and frustrated by the people they served in the name of the Lord.

The eminent missionary scholar Arthur H. Smith (1845–1932) wrote that "The Chinese are not naturally a religious people. Although to the superficial observer they appear very religious ... on closer examination it is evident that most of their worship is empty formalism. While the Hindus are passionately fond of the metaphysical and speculative, the Chinese are practical and do not burden themselves with the mysteries of the invisible world." One of the reasons that Leonora, rather than Alex, was so successful in her work was evinced by Smith, who echoed the opinions of missionaries the world over in his statement that "... the women are the most devout worshippers: many of the educated men are skeptics, making only an outward acknowledgement of forms of worship."[4]

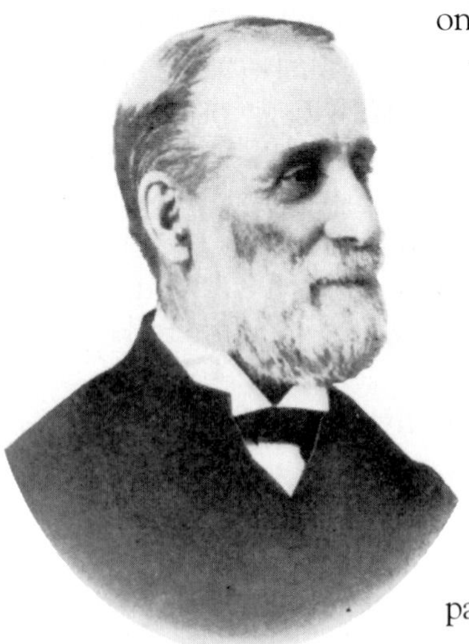

Famed missionary Dr. Arthur H. Smith

The four great old religions of China were the ethical (Confucianism), the physical (Taoism), the metaphysical (Buddhism), and as a combination of all three, Ancestor Worship. Other faiths, almost unrecognizable after centuries of assimilation, were Islam and Judaism, although Muslim Chinese did not marry outside their faith. One reason that all four major religions survived, in fact coexisted, was a pragmatic approach on the part of the Chinese to the role of religion in general. The upheavals, including torture, war, and mass genocide that accompanied the development of other religions did not take place in China. For millennia the Chinese had considered their world to be an entity unto itself, populated by one great human family ruled by one sovereign, the Emperor, or the Son of Heaven. China, as the "centre of the world," was called the Middle Kingdom, and it was quite happy to remain unmoved by the rest of the world. All religions, including, finally, Christianity, were allowed to coexist — provided they did not upset the Chinese way of life.

In the very old days, primitive religions considered the observable and the supernatural as merely separate expressions of the same phenomenon. By the late 19th century the Chinese were still largely indifferent to doctrinal conflicts. Religious feeling was more a reflection of the harmony of nature: religious rites and practices were means of enhancing and preserving this harmony. By the time Leonora and Alex arrived on the scene, Buddhism had adopted the deities and spirits of other religions; Taoism had imitated the trinity of Buddhism, and according to American missionary Dr. Martin, Confucianism despised, rejected, and yet adopted both. Every Chinese, reported Martin, was a Confucianist, but "most of them are likewise Taoists and Buddhists. They practise all three on different occasions and for different purposes." Arthur H. Smith added that there was, in fact, no Chinese word that embodied the concept of religion — the closest phrase, *p'ai shên*, meant, approximately, "to worship," or to pay one's respects to gods and spirits. This was, he wrote, "a vague substitute for a word which should mean religion."

One of the problems that Alex would face was that Confucius, adapting works by the earlier Mencius, never taught duty to a power any higher than the head of state, or indeed of family. The Emperor, being the Son of Heaven, had a direct line and was, in fact, the only person allowed to worship Heaven (rather than a God). This he did each year at the two solstices, in the soaring, magnificent Temple of Heaven in Peking, having first fasted, meditated, and prepared with an elaborate and solemn ceremonial process. The closest that the Emperor's worship would come to Christianity — in this case Catholicism — would lie in accepting blame, or confessing sins under, say, circumstances of drought, flood or pestilence, for which disasters he and he alone was responsible.

Viceroy Li Hung-chang said that having read the New Testament (presumably in Chinese), he saw very little difference between its teachings and those of Confucianism, and this, wrote Arthur Smith, was probably the professed attitude of many Confucianists. Li's fellow Viceroy Chang Chih-tung noted that "The higher class of Chinese should carefully consider the situation and should tolerate the Western Religion as they tolerate Buddhism and Taoism. Why should it injure us? And because Confucianism, as now practised, is inadequate to lift us from the present plight (that of a crumbling, insular empire), why retaliate by scoffing at other religions?" Not only was such a procedure useless, wrote the Viceroy, but it was, in fact, rather dangerous.

In an elaborate essay read at the World's Parliament of Religions in the last century, a Mr. P'ung remarked that, to a Confucianist, Christianity in China was devoid of interest. "Mr. P'ung complains, as in view of its contrast to the minuteness of the Book of Rites he well might, that the New Testament directions for social conduct are very meager. Confucianism has been very carefully studied by Western scholars, and its excellence and its defects have been thoroughly presented. If at a former period there was an excess of antagonism ... on the part of some missionaries, there is now a tendency to a wholesome reaction, and it is regarded rather in the light of a preparation for Christianity." The issue of contention, apparently, was an irreconcilable opposition regarding ancestor worship.[5]

Another viceroy, Tuan Fang, remarked: "We take pleasure in bearing testimony to the part taken by American missionaries in promoting the progress of the Chinese people. They have borne the light of Western civilization into every nook and corner of the empire. The awaking of China ... may be traced in no small measure to the hands of the missionaries. For this service you will find China not ungrateful." There were others, however, who would disagree vehemently.

As a missionary physician Leonora would have had to juggle her own religious beliefs, not only with her

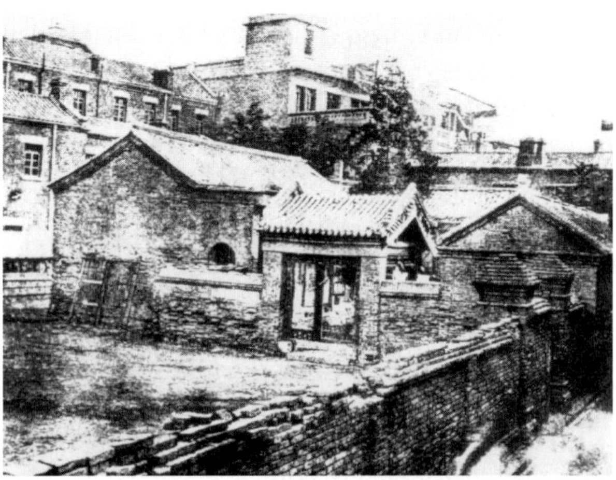

Lady Li and Leonora's hospital in Tientsin

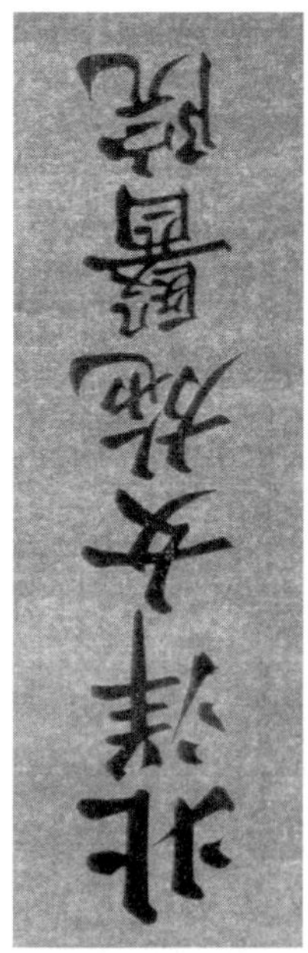

Government Hospital for Women and Children

Chinese benefactors and patients, but also with her colleagues. Leonora, Alex and a number of other missionaries were hard-working and compassionate people. There were, however, others who held the Chinese in lower esteem, and seemed more determined to save souls than bodies. Not the least of these was Leonora's successor at the Isabella Fisher Hospital, Dr. L.E. Akers.

Dr. Akers started her service in good spirits, spending her first year doing little but learning Chinese. But she quickly developed a sharply critical view of the Chinese. In April 1884, she and Elizabeth Yates embarked on a trip to the outstations of Chihli Province. Whether or not it was the latter's influence that soured Dr. Akers is unknown, but the reports of both women were unusually blunt. Miss Yates wrote that although she was "especially encouraged" in revisiting the section she had seen the previous winter, "Sometimes in those lonely days it seemed ... that the 'line upon line and precept upon precept' made no impression whatever upon the callous consciences and benighted minds about me. My heart did realize something of the joyful reaping that follows tearful sowing ... people were standing upon a higher plane ... because of my efforts, though made in much weakness."

Poor Dr. Akers did not enjoy her first field trip, and she was one of the few WFMS members to complain publicly, rather than lamenting strictly to family and friends. "[It] did our hearts and souls good, but was rather hard physically ... I was thirteen hours in the saddle, while Miss Yates was jolted over rough roads in a flat bottomed cart, without springs. When we reached our inn ... we were too tired to think of supper ... Miss Yates nibbled a bit of dry cake, while I appeased my long-empty stomach on a fossil biscuit and piece of cold mutton; meanwhile dragging my stiffening limbs back and forth ... fearing to go to bed ... less the morning should find me too unwilling to mount for the home stretch."

Although Leonora was still in charge of medical work at Tientsin during 1884, Dr. Akers gradually took over and as she did so, the tone of the Isabella Fisher Hospital, and the Dispensary, began to change. Where Leonora Howard King was universally regarded as gentle and loving toward Chinese women and children, Dr. Akers had different ideas. "We have felt," she wrote, "for a long time, that more than we were doing must be done ... so we have put the little organ into one of the rooms in the Dispensary, and every morning as the patients come they are put in this room to wait. Miss Yates sings, and talks and prays ... I call them by a bell to my room ... and treat them for the bodily ailments. Poor things! They are so fearfully stupid and blind with all their sinfulness ... The times of refreshing by sight are comparatively few here." In the next report Miss Yates called the Chinese women "blind and ignorant," and Akers called them "suffering, stupid creatures," and "wretched."

Dr. Akers was not alone in her distaste for the Chinese. Missionary dentist Reverend R.H. Graves wrote, regarding Britain's shameful opium war attack of 1840–1842, that "I have heard Chinese, in other respects intelligent, speak of the war of the English against China as "rebellion," and foreigners who oppose the will of the Emperor as "rebels." It was not strange, he went on to say, that "a people whose self-conceit is so marked should cling to the traditions of the past and be slow to yield the palm of superiority to any other nation." Graves, who called the Chinese "profoundly ignorant" also noted that "Just as some conceited heathen [presumably the aforementioned Mr. P'ung] went away from the Parliament of Religions in Chicago with the notion that Americans are getting tired of Christianity and sought them as religious instructions ... so these Chinese ... have jumped at the conclusion that ... scholars are trying to introduce Confucianism into Europe."[6]

Canadian Reverend James Frazer Smith, himself a physician, complained that after the Chinese had performed their temple worship, they left in a "noisy and flippant" manner. "Worship performed in such a spirit ... is of no real benefit," intoned the doctor/churchman. Although Frazer Smith was fairly indulgent toward the Chinese, he also recounts amazingly heroic instances of holding off hordes of rioters with the mere impressiveness of his demeanour and by "haranguing the throng" into well-behaved believing.[7]

But Alex and Leonora were in a way unusual for their time: later missionaries emulated their way of life, concentrating more on healing the sick, teaching hygiene and preventive medicine than dwelling on conversion, and, in Alex's case, preaching the case of a gentle God rather than a force that would terrorize the Chinese people into submission.

In the meantime, Leonora and Alex began to set up housekeeping. It is unlikely that Leonora's house-cum-dispensary would have been deemed adequate for a Western couple, especially with the frantic race for social prestige that was rampant in China's port cities. Dr. George "Chinese" Morrison put it succinctly, much to the dismay of those who felt they should be portrayed as "roughing it." Morrison, book author and correspondent for *The Times*, had a marvellous habit of using biting sarcasm in his literary efforts. In his 1895 book, *An Australian in China*, he often took potshots at China missionaries, and seemed to enjoy it thoroughly. "Among the most comfortable residences are missionary quarters," he asserted, "and it is but right that the missionaries should be separated as far as possible from all discomfort — missionaries who are sacrificing all for China, and who are prepared to undergo any reasonable hardship to bring enlightenment to this land of darkness." Under most circumstances, and indeed in the case of Dr. Leonora Howard King and her churchman husband, Morrison was, quite truthfully, right on the button.

It was generally accepted, albeit at great cost in Chinese labour, that missionaries would transport Western beds, stoves, pianos, dishes and endless bric-a-brac ordered from Montgomery Ward's catalogue through the tortuous peaks, valleys, canals and rivers of China. Although he was later to be unmasked as a rogue, Morrison related what he saw as the truth. But this type of criticism would seldom affect even the most stalwart Servant of God.

Missionary gardens were both beautiful and useful. Some women took pride in counting exactly how many blossoms or bushes they had grown: one lady counted 249 rose blossoms, and another had 89 rose bushes alone. But most women, including Leonora, worked with their servants to create gardens that were also functional. Leonora and Alex's mansion in Tientsin included camellias, azaleas and wisteria, perhaps peonies, calla lilies, hyacinths and irises in springtime; roses, daisies, hydrangeas in the summer, and dahlias and chrysanthemums in fall. Peach, pear, apple and plum blossoms rioted in spring, and grape vines provided shade throughout the summer. Most important though, by supervising the cultivation of her own vegetables, Leonora could ensure that any "night-soil" (fertilizer) used would be animal, rather than human, waste.

The Kings' home was spacious and airy, with numerous Chinese ornaments and elegant chairs — a far cry from other missionary homes that, wrote one American, "lookt shoddy because they were furnisht with ... odds and ends brought from America: the owners had not had individuality or enterprise enuf

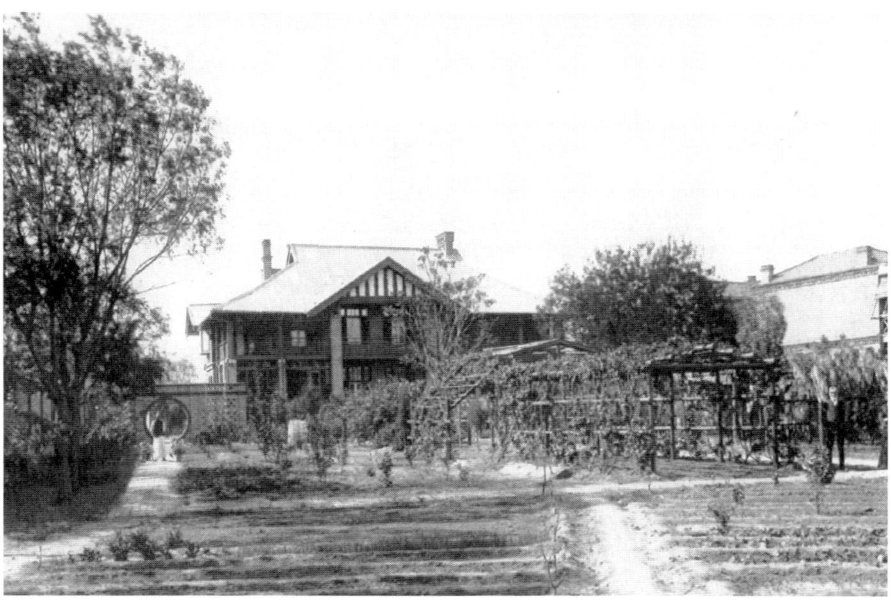

The back garden with moon-gate

to look around them, discover the products that China excells in and utilize them ... ."[8] Although their living quarters contained a few pieces of Canadian furniture — notably a writing desk now converted to a display table, a butler's table, fine lace curtains and a leopard-skin-covered easy chair, Leonora and Alex were exceptions to the rule of rarely using Chinese objets d'art in their homes. Porcelain and silver vases, bowls and pretty Chinese tea sets graced the living room, and a delicate embroidered screen shielded the fireplace in summertime. Tientsin was known for its exquisite carpets, and their floor was covered wall-to-wall with a beautifully detailed, hand-woven product. Although many other missionary women purchased statuary, lace, lacquers, paintings and embroidery, most things of beauty were sent home to Mother. As a result of this common action, "Chinoiserie" collecting became the rage for a number of years, particularly in English and North American Victorian-style homes.

The Kings' home in Tientsin was, by any standards, a mansion. Three stories high, it was decidedly British in character, right down to some black-and-white Tudor stripes. Huge pillars gave a rather heavy dignity to the whole structure, but a note of grace and serendipity was added through the addition of round Chinese "moon-gates" at the walled compound's entrance. Spacious, airy verandahs encircled the house on two floors, and over the years English ivy or Virginia creeper would lend a homey atmosphere. Good solid maple trees,

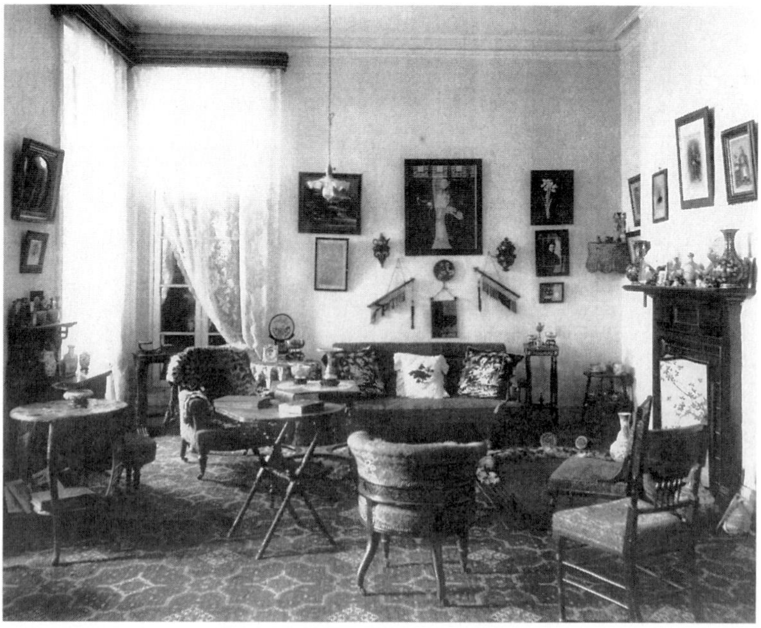

The Kings' drawing room, Tientsin

reminiscent of Leonora's Canadian heritage (but also indigenous to China), would grow large and provide welcome shade for the couple's later years. Within the high Chinese-style walled compound one did not find an equally Chinese courtyard, but a Canadian-style lawn dotted with fruit trees. Beyond the lawn, row upon row of vegetables and herbs flourished in the mild coastal climate. Although the house was more Western than Chinese in architecture, the Kings did not have the dubious taste of one Canadian missionary who had an enormous Union Jack incorporated into his roof tiles.[9]

By the early 1880s, Tientsin's foreign community had set firm social standards for hiring servants. The minimum number was three: cook, houseboy and coolie, and being a woman, Leonora would already have a "mafoo" or general factotum to ensure her safety on the road. An amah, of course, would take care of any children, though Leonora and Alex would remain childless, and a gardener was de rigueur. In justification for this seeming ostentation, each household had to do for itself what was normally done by a whole community back home. One had to supply sewer, garbage and transportation services, as well as one's own health system, which included the ubiquitous vegetable garden and fruit orchard. With no telephones a coolie was necessary, for all foreigners adopted the British system of sending "chits," or written messages, between home, office, church or hospital. Finally, as the missionaries prospered, entertaining long-term house guests and holding banquets became the norm. By the time Leonora and Alex King retired, they would have 10 servants to run a two-person household.*

Medical facilities followed suit. Viceroy Li Hung-chang, recognizing the limitations of a small, rather dark former temple, had now built John Kenneth Mackenzie a proper hospital of his own. Lady Li, not to be outdone, followed suit on Leonora's behalf. Leonora's newest hospital was, in fact, another "first" for the Canadian doctor, being the first hospital for women and children built entirely with Chinese funds. *The Daily News*, published out of Shanghai, reported that "The new hospital buildings in the [Tientsin] settlement are making rapid progress. They will [cost] $2,000, much of which is already subscribed to by the Chinese. Many prominent officials manifest an interest in this enterprise. The medical work for women under the care of Miss Dr. Howard is in a like flourishing condition. A permanent building will soon be erected for its accommodation.

"We have here as the outgrowth of Christianity and of Christian Missions a spectacle such as it not to be found elsewhere in China, viz., two large institutes,

*Letter from a member of the Howard family.

side-by-side, for ministering to the diseased and the destitute. One, under the care of Dr. Mackenzie [sic], built and supported by funds contributed by the Chinese, is for men only; the other, under the care of Dr. Howard, and built by funds from one of the lands of the west, reaches out its healing mercies to the women and children of China." This latter reference should actually have referred to Lady Li's new hospital, but record keepers of the times often confused facts and dates. "Both are under the patronage of the Viceroy Li and his excellent Countess — himself one of the highest and most enlightened of Chinese officials."[10]

Leonora's impact on Li Hung-chang, his family and his subjects cannot be underestimated. A plaque presented to her by Li, saying "A doctor is interested in curing people, not in profit," now graced the portals of her new hospital. It is a matter of record that Li meant what he said. Part of a speech that he later made to American missionaries repeated this philosophy. "The missionaries have not sought for pecuniary gain at the hands of our people. They have not been secret emissaries of diplomatic schemes. Their labors have no political significance, and last, but not least, if I might be permitted to add, they have not interfered with or usurped the rights of territorial authorities. A man is composed of soul, intellect, and body. I highly appreciate that your eminent Boards (Foreign Missionary Boards of the United States) in your arduous and most esteemed work in China, have neglected none of the three."[11]

Overseas, in Leonora's native Canada, the Student Volunteer Movement that had swept the United States began to be felt throughout the land. In 1880, more than 1,800 Canadian and United States students had declared that they were "willing and desirous, God permitting, to be Foreign Missionaries." Divinity students began asking themselves whether it was right to spend a lifetime competing with other ministers for the "privilege of preaching to a comparatively small group ... who already enjoy all the advantages of a Christian community."[12]

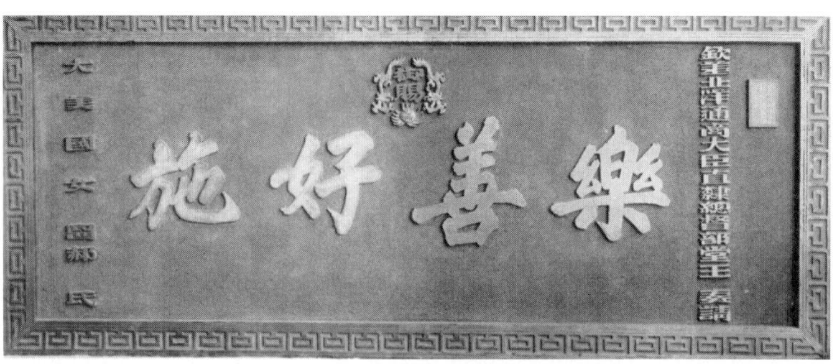

Li's gift to Leonora

The answer was invariably negative, since in Canada funds were lacking for any but the most simple posting to lumber camp or Indian reserve. In a rising tide of enthusiasm at Queen's University — the institution that had denied Leonora her medical studies — young people decided to raise funds to send their own volunteers overseas. At the regular gathering of the University Missionary Association on January 30, 1886, discussion became so intense that it continued through three successive meetings. Finally a resolution would pledge continued support for home missions, but also support a foreign mission of the students' own. An appeal was made to all students, to former members of the missionary association, and to all Queen's graduates. The response, though not as liberal as expected, was encouraging enough that the students redoubled their fund-raising efforts.

Young James Frazer Smith, a medical and divinity student at Queen's, found himself posted for three months at St. Mark's Church in Toronto. Residing for the time being at Knox College, he met up with equally young Jonathan Goforth, "a very zealous theological student, and most enthusiastic about Foreign missions." Between the two of them, the eager students formed a similar foreign mission scheme at Knox College. In November Frazer Smith, as President of the Queen's Missionary Association, stated his case for going out to China. His fellow students responded to the offer "with deep emotion," and a few weeks later, by unanimous vote, it was "*Resolved:* ... That Mr. J. Frazer Smith, who has offered himself to the Lord and to this Association for work in the Foreign field, be appointed the first Foreign Missionary of Queen's University Missionary Association." A similar resolution from Knox College adopted fire-and-brimstone Goforth.

Like Leonora Howard these young men were, for their last years at school, sponsored by the missionary associations. A delighted Frazer Smith wrote "that my great desire to go to work Abroad as a thoroughly qualified medical missionary, with extra special courses added, was in this providential way to be gratified." It would be impossible, he said, to describe the feeling of freedom he experienced "on being so wonderfully released from the burden of the financial anxieties, in connection with the completion of my medical course." Two years later, on January 24, 1888, Dr. James Frazer Smith was ordained a church minister, and designated by the presbytery of Kingston as a missionary "for work in Honan, China, a province of over twenty millions of people." Like Alex King, Frazer Smith would need a wife in the field, and on April 18 he married Miss Minnie Waugh of Hamilton, Ontario, a lady "devoted in the cause of Foreign Missions."

At the Queen's University convocation, the students, who had among them raised almost $800 for the Frazer Smiths' travel and medical supplies rose as one to sing:

"From Greenland's icy mountains,
From India's coral strand,
Where Africa's sunny fountains
Roll down their golden sand,
From many an ancient river,
From many a palmy plain,
They call us to deliver
Their land from error's chain."[13]

Honan Province had been chosen because it was second only to Hunan in being the most hostile province to foreigners, but also because Americans, British, French, Swedish and German missionaries had already laid claim to other areas. Dr. Hudson Taylor, founder of the China Inland Mission, remarked to the Canadians, "If your missionaries ever succeed in locating in Honan, it will only be as they go forward on their knees." And so, at least figuratively speaking, it would be.

Frazer Smith and his wife would remain in Canada so that he could complete his medical degree. It was, therefore, Jonathan Goforth and his wife who arrived as the first official[14] Canadian missionaries in China. The proposed party of four — two missionaries, two wives — was then increased by Miss Harriet R. Sutherland, a graduate nurse, who represented the new [Canadian] Women's Missionary Society. She would be the first official — rather than spousal — Canadian missionary woman in China. By the end of August 1888, the five young people were "settled temporarily" at Chefoo, North China, and the two men were "most anxious" to make a tour of inspection several hundred miles inland.

Like many other newcomers, they were in for a big disappointment. They were "greatly surprised" to learn that it was impossible to travel for any distance, or even to work by themselves without a knowledge of either Chinese language or customs. Finally a tour was arranged through the kind offers of Arthur H. Smith and the Reverend F.M. Chapin, who would accompany as interpreters and protectors. Goforth and Frazer Smith travelled by steamer to Tientsin, where they were entertained by Dr. and Mrs. Stanley of the American Board. It is very likely that, as the first Canadian missionaries, they would also have met with Leonora and Alex. Who knows what the fundamentalist Goforth must have thought of the city dwellers' palatial homes and modern facilities?

A man of some wit, Frazer Smith later remembered the dreaded Peking carts by writing:

Let those who vote Lake Como "slow"
Or grumble on the banks of Po
And wonder where they next can go,
Try a cart ride on the plains of Chili [sic].

The doctor also quipped that the squeaking noise of ungreased wheels, which carried all over the plains for miles, "must be heard in order to be appreciated … . The Chinese inn is not to be pictured but tested," and, speaking of accommodations at such inns, "Your couch becomes a hunting ground, Where rats and smaller game abound."

In 1888, the Yellow River, or "China's Sorrow," had once more flooded its banks. In Honan, where Frazer Smith and Goforth were headed, destruction, desolation, death and disease reigned supreme, but without knowledge of the language the new arrivals could not render much assistance. This latest breach in the Yellow River was the site of many Chinese attempts to close the gap — with the traditional bundling of "scores of tons" of kaoliange stalks — similar to cornstalks but stronger — then rebundling the small bundles into huge heaps with strong rope, cemented with clay and weighted with stones. Foreign engineers had, in fact, been consulted by the Chinese, but their methods were felt to be too costly. Frazer Smith wrote that "hopeless as the task appeared, patience, and perseverance, noted characteristics of the Chinese … won the day."

As 1888 drew to a close, two more Canadians arrived in Chefoo. They were Dr. William McClure, a graduate and gold medallist from McGill University in Montreal, and Reverend Donald MacGillivray, another gold medallist from the University of Toronto. Within a few months McClure had married Margaret Baird of the American Presbyterian Mission, Canton. During the summer Harriet Sutherland married the Rev. Dr. Hunter Corbett of Chefoo, and like Leonora Howard with the WFMS, she left the Canadian contingent for her husband's organization, the American Presbyterian Board. In December 1889, eight new workers arrived. They included the Reverends John MacDougall, John Harvey MacVicar, and Murdoch MacKenzie and their wives, and two graduate nurses, Margaret McIntosh and Jeanie Graham.

With blithe self-assurance the "Honan Presbytery," with Goforth as Moderator, decided to settle in the two prefectural cities of Changte and Weihwei. Little did they know, wrote Frazer Smith, of the "many changes that would take place, or of the patient and strenuous effort … nor … owing to the bitter and determined opposition of the people, some years of anxious struggle would elapse before their fond hopes of occupying these chosen centres would be realized."

Thus, 15 Canadian missionaries spent almost two years in "the enormous daily grind at the language," being entirely supported by the financial contributions of the good folks at home. In 1890, the men finally rented two houseboats, each containing a clerical member and a physician, and, much to their relief, Christian Chinese assistants loaned from other missions. An "ample supply of medicines and instruments ... and a full assortment of Christian literature in Chinese, both for sale and for free distribution," was taken on each boat. Although the missionaries set up shop in Chinese inns, renting one room for preaching and the other for a doctor's dispensary, they demurred at the thought of occupying these rooms at night, preferring to live on the houseboats. It was evident, reported Dr. Frazer Smith, that a long and bitter struggle would ensue before a location would be secured in any of the chief cities.

The group finally proceeded along the path of least resistance, locating their missions in smaller towns. Aside from flat defiance on the part of city officials, people at home were wondering what was happening to all their money. There was, said Frazer Smith, "the urge from the Home Church, the members of which, as the months went by, were waiting to hear ... that their missionaries had at length settled in Honan." Of course the missionaries themselves were eager to show the Chinese that they had come to do them good. In summer 1890, Dr. McClure and Mr. MacGillivray moved into a compound in Chu Wang. For awhile the two men, keeping a low profile, managed to make some inroads. Then one day a deputation of "friendly neighbours" paid a call. After some "complimentary speeches," and the necessary derogatory remarks about their own poor town and its residents, the deputation politely suggested that the missionaries move on to another place "more worthy of their distinguished talents." A few days later, several hundred men rushed the compound and carried off "instruments, medicines, books, bedding and clothing," not even leaving "a cup to drink from." The idea was that when McClure and MacGillivray left to purchase new supplies, they would be barred from re-entering the town. The doctor wrote, "Little did they realize the manner of men they were dealing with."

At the time, Goforth and Frazer Smith were a few miles away on a houseboat tour. A coolie sent to deliver a bundle of mail to McClure and MacGillivray returned with a scrap of paper reading "Come, we want you. McClure." The Chinese were, apparently, in a state of consternation at the appearance of two more of the Foreign Devils. Where had they come from? A rumour was spread that since telegraphic communications had now been established between Tientsin and Tai Ming Fu, both in Chihli province, the newcomers had simply been sent by telegraph to Tai Ming Fu (some 96 kilometres away) and that the wind had blown them the rest of the way. Owing to the cool weather, Frazer Smith arrived dressed in a fine maroon coloured dressing gown and a black knitted lounging cap. This, he wrote, together with his physical stature, seemed to designate him as leader of the foreign party. As the costume went over so well with the Chinese, the doctor would use it to impress Chinese officials for many years, to the amusement of his fellow missionaries.

Finally a "weak and worthless" proclamation was issued and a few stolen things returned, with a Chinese shrug that nothing further could be done on the Canadians' behalf. Goforth decided to appeal to Li Hung-chang through the British Consul at Tientsin. Li issued strict orders to settle the case with full compensation for all the missing goods, two proclamations guaranteeing full protection were issued, and a peace banquet, of "thirty six bowls, some nine different courses," was paid for by the district Mandarin and "outwardly at least" the populace was a little more friendly.

There is no record of Leonora's having to endure the ire and hostility of Chinese mobs. Although some female missionaries would be harassed, even murdered in years to come, it was the men, not the women, who were considered a threat by the Chinese. It is easy to imagine Chinese reaction to these huge, gruff, bearded creatures, who simply made bold decisions to settle in their midst and attempt to change their whole way of life. Itinerant women like Leonora, who were considered beneath notice by Chinese society, were usually received, if not warmly, with interest. Leonora cured and preached, then moved on. She, with her "long nose" and huge feet, held no physical attraction to Chinese men. But in a China where many men had more than one wife, male missionaries might be construed as a threat to Chinese women.

Another Canadian property was secured in Hsin Chen, about 100 kilometres from the Chu Wang compound. Like most properties the early missionaries took over, this one was fairly filthy, had rickety doors, small windows, and mud or brick floors. At first, in order not to give offence, the Canadians merely changed the doors and windows, laid a board floor on the brick, put new straw mats on the ceilings, and scraped and whitewashed the walls. One day a beggar-band calling themselves "The Blood Spilling Guild" rushed the compound, "brandishing their knives ... faces and hands smeared with their own blood." Their objective apparently was to terrorize the missionaries into giving them as much money as possible, with a view to future investments. MacGillivray, who had from the beginning adopted Chinese dress and hairstyle, was dragged about the yard by his queue. MacVicar was knocked about and threatened with long knives. Nothing much came of it, although the two stood side by side for five hours holding the mob at bay. Some Chinese "friends" advised them to go into hiding. They refused, wisely, it turned out, as shortly thereafter two Swedish missionaries who had taken similar advice were dragged from their hiding place and "brained."

Dr. Frazer Smith had been away in Lin Ching. His return trip with fellow missionary MacDougall had been speedy, owing to a favourable tail wind. The doctor wrote that on his arrival MacGillivray exclaimed "Thank God you have come! You have saved us!" After an accusation that the missionaries had killed one of the beggars — Frazer Smith tapped the beggar on a "very responsive" part to determine that the beggar was quite alive. He then apparently dispersed the huge crowd by shaking his walking stick and berating the Chinese in a loud voice. "I took command," said the doctor, and miraculously the beggar king returned with all the missionaries' silver nuggets.[15]

The Canadian women, Frazer Smith's wife in particular, had a rougher time of it than did Leonora, protected by Li Hung-chang in the cosmopolitan centre of Tientsin. During the aforementioned debacle, Mrs. Smith had lost an infant son to acute dysentery. During that first winter in the field she must have been terribly lonely, being the only foreign woman at Hsin Chen. She and her remaining child, "Cammie," were, like Leonora and the other female missionaries, the source of much curiosity among Chinese women and children. "Crowds of women and children," wrote her husband, "clamoured at the gate to see the foreign lady and the little boy. Forty to fifty ... a day was a small average."

There was another difference between Leonora's and Frazer Smith's experiences, again having to do with taking over Chinese property, rather than being a travelling preacher. The inland missionaries kept themselves barricaded inside their walled properties simply to avoid disease. At times, he wrote, mothers carrying children recovering from smallpox were "refused admission." This could only serve to alienate the rural populace, who had been told they would be welcome to hear the strange teachings — and be healed by — these Foreign Devils. With this type of selective soul-saving, it is little wonder that the Honan missionaries endured so many hostile mobbings including, wrote the doctor, one during a period where little Cammie was seriously ill with malaria. One small comfort for Mrs. Smith and her son, and for many other women in the field, was a pet dog.

"Women's work" was highly prized by the Canadians. Out of three original nurses, only Margaret McIntosh made it inland. A plea was sent home to Canada for "another single lady, preferably a physician," and in fall of 1892, 15 years after Leonora Howard had arrived in Peking, Dr. Lucinda Graham, recently graduated from the new Women's Medical College in Toronto, would arrive "to great rejoicing."[16] She was the second Canadian woman doctor in China.

War clouds were gathering yet again, this time with the threat of Japanese invasion of another tributary country, Korea. Writing from the Isabella Fisher Hospital, Elizabeth Yates wrote: "You will be feeling very anxious about us, but I assure you that we are in no danger personally ... . All this may be just what is needed in bringing this selfish, covetous nation to a better understanding of their own weakness."

Endnotes

1. Council for World Missionary Archives, Day Missions Library, Yale University. London Missionary Society Records. Box H-2139. 1885.
2. Ibid.
3. Goodall, N. A *History of the London Missionary Society, 1895-1945*. London: Oxford University Press, 1954, p. 168.
4. Smith, Arthur H. *The Uplift of China*. New York: Forward Mission Study Courses. Young People's Missionary Movement, 1907, p. 85.
5. Ibid., p. 99.
6. Graves, R.H. *Forty Years in China*. Baltimore, Maryland: R.H. Woodward Company, 1895, pp. 39-40.
7. Frazer Smith, James, Reverend, MD, CM. *Life's Waking Part*. Toronto: Thomas Nelson and Sons Limited, 1937, pp. 166-169.
8. Hunter, Jane. *The Gospel of Gentility - American Women Missionaries in Turn-of-the-Century China*. New Haven: Yale University Press, 1984, p. 134.
9. Victoria College, University of Toronto. Presbyterian Church in Canada. Board of Foreign Missions Fonds. Records Pertaining to the Honan Mission, 1887-1937. Reference 122/6/1. Reverend Murdoch MacKenzie's home, Changte, Honan Province.
10. *Chinese Recorder* 11, p. 310.
11. Speech by Li Hung-chang, quoted in Smith, Arthur H., *Uplift of China*, p. 116.
12. Frazer Smith, *Life's Waking Part*, p. 65.
13. Ibid., pp. 68-72.
14. Remember, Leonora Howard King was sent out by the American Methodist Episcopal Society's Woman's Foreign Missionary Society.
15. Frazer Smith, *Life's Walking Part*, pp. 146-155.
16. Ibid., p. 197.

Chapter fifteen

Modernizing China
1887–1894

"...the lack of men of ability in the court is really ridiculous."
— Li Hung-chang

Tientsin was on the road to modernization, with much of the credit going to Li Hung-chang himself. New construction was sweeping the old port city, and Leonora not only had a modern, well-equipped hospital, but she could also stroll through lovely Victoria Park, a "whites' only"* oasis of rose gardens across from the newly constructed Astor House Hotel. Because the construction had attracted many foreigners, someone had to accommodate them while their own magnificent homes were being built. The hotel and the rose gardens, as part of an English-Chinese partnership, were the brainchild of George Gustav Detring, a German-born British subject who had entered into many other construction projects with Li Hung-chang.

Although Tientsin was the major gateway to Peking, the roadway to that city was, until 1887, a rough dirt track that became a sea of mud on rainy days and impassable in times of flood. This 500 year-old irritation would now be rectified, again by Leonora's mentor and his Western business associates. Both Westerners and Chinese investors, having had experience in building other stone roads, took a vote on improving this all-important route. They quickly collected 1,600 taels of silver and began to hire labourers and collect stones from outlying fields. After several months of construction, the road between Tientsin and Yangcun, a town between Tientsin and Peking, was completed. It would not be repaired until 1949.

---

*Li Hung-chang and his family were exceptions.

The North China Mission of the WFMS now had five full-time workers, including two more women physicians. One newer arrival, Nellie R. Green, wrote that "China seems moving as she has never done before, and 'Western' influence is impressing itself on the whole land in such a way that sooner or later the darkness must recede before the light. Not only direct missionary effort, but social and secular power is making itself felt. The outlook is encouraging or discouraging, as one turns toward the light, or toward the darkness, it is right to keep well both in mind, that we may work to the best advantage … ."

The missionaries still became ill with alarming frequency. If they were not felled by typhoid, cholera or malaria, their eyes often gave out as a result of too much paperwork. Many went to Japan for a rest, rather than sailing all the way home, but others like Leonora and Alex retreated during the hottest months to mountain temples and seaside resorts. Dr. Anna D. Gloss, who had taken over from Dr. Akers at the Isabella Fisher Hospital, reported carefully that, "It was a great trial for me to close the hospital for a month at this season when we have so many patients, but as it is easier to *keep* well than to *get* well in China, I yielded to the advice of my friends." Dr. Gloss, while excusing her own behaviour, hastened to return to the missionary business at hand, not without taking a sly poke at Leonora's defection from the WFMS. "The new hospital built in the neighbourhood of ours, by Lady Li for Dr. Howard King, is now completed and will doubtless be opened this autumn," she said. "The last shadow of this lady's patronage departed from us when a month since Mrs. King sent for the 'piero' which had been presented by Lady Li at the opening of the Isabella Fisher Hospital, and has since then adorned our front entrance." Dr. Gloss may have been masking some envy when she continued, "Of course, most of the official patronage goes with Mrs. King, but there is plenty of work among the poorer classes, and if I did not feel that the ladies at home would be greatly disappointed, I should feel rather relieved than otherwise to be free from a service so enslaving, and which bears so little fruit for Christ."

Anna Gloss may be forgiven for feeling slighted under the circumstances, as much as Leonora may be forgiven for taking whatever she could get from the Chinese, rather than the tight-fisted missionary societies. "Lady Li's interest has always been personal and has never been transferred in the least degree to the mission — or to Mrs. King's successors," wrote Dr. Gloss indignantly. "Her influence was doubtless of great importance when the work was first started, but we can have plenty of work to-day without her."[1]

For all the benefits of Westernization, a tragic pall still cast itself over millions of Chinese homes. Leonora's new hospital would of necessity have a separate ward for treating opium addicts. Patients were on the whole still healthy and well fed, and could afford to pay in silver to kick the habit. They had yet to be reduced to the vacant-eyed, ragged ghosts who had sold all their possessions, dispossessed their families, reneged on their debts and now pitifully begged former colleagues for funds to support their addiction. One of Leonora's main problems was that patients in the first stages of addiction often absconded with anything movable for "just one more smoke" — after all, one more wouldn't do them any harm, and the long-nosed lady doctor could certainly afford to replace any item stolen.

Tientsin, like most other Chinese cities, abounded in shops that sold opium-smoking paraphernalia, and every bank, silk shop and hong [warehouse-office] had an opium-room with the lamp lit for honoured guests. Even the Empress Dowager was known to indulge — as Queen Victoria still puffed on the odd cigarette — but it was well known that Tz'u-hsi would never become a soulless wreck lying in the gutter. Since she had lost both a husband and a son to this and other types of debauchery, the Empress's own use of opium was infrequent.

In 1893, 4,275 tons of Indian opium was imported to China, courtesy of the British.[2] Although Li Hung-chang publicly condemned the drug, pragmatists found it difficult to believe he was sincere. Li was, in fact, far more opposed to the *importation* of foreign opium, and therefore the profits made by the British, than to the drug itself. Back in 1881, Li had sent a letter to Reverend F. Storrs Turner, secretary of the Society for the Suppression of the Opium Trade, admitting, in part, that "the poppy is certainly surreptitiously grown in some parts of China, notwithstanding the laws and frequent Imperial edicts prohibiting its cultivation." He continued "I earnestly hope that your Society, and all right-minded men of your country, will support the efforts China is now making to escape from the thraldom of opium." But rumour had it that Li's own family continued to make enormous profits from cultivating the poppy. At the Missionary Conference of 1888, The Reverend G. Piercy said "... China has not done with the evils of opium, even if our hands were washed of this traffic to-day. China in her desperation has invoked Satan to chase out Satan. She now grows her own opium, vainly dreaming that, if the Indian supply lapse, she can then deal with this rapidly growing evil."[3]

A petition, signed "spontaneously" by thousands of Chinese (via the missionaries) was now circulated both in China and abroad by the Society for the Suppression of Opium Trade. It read, in part: "Some tens of millions of human beings in distress are looking on tiptoe with outstretched necks for salvation to come from you, O just and benevolent men of England! If not for the good or honour of your country, then for mercy's sake do this good deed now to save a people, and the rescued millions shall ... be your great reward."[4] One official who had been a government inspector of opium manufacturing in India had felt so keenly the guilt of his share in the traffic that he contributed the savings of his official career, amounting to over $3,000, for the relief of opium sufferers in China.[5] His gesture, though admirable, was in vain.

Opium was regarded by merchants in the same way a tot of good whisky might oil the wheels of a lucrative business deal, and edicts against the drug were usually drawn up by Chinese philanthropists over a quiet pipe of opium, signed by opium-smoking officials whose revenues were derived from the poppy, and posted near fields of poppy by the opium-smoking magistrates who owned them. Morbid tales of "lank and shrivelled limbs, tottering gait, sallow visage, feeble voice, and death-boding glance of eye"[6] continued to fill missionaries' reports home, but in all truth Leonora may have seldom seen such far-gone misery. This may well have been because they went away to die in private, or because the vast majority of Chinese who could afford the drug were only moderately addicted and seemed, like English "Opium Eater" Thomas de Quincy, to remain at a comfortable plateau.

Leonora would, however, frequently have treated Chinese wives for opium overdoses. This was a particularly popular method of suicide, being easy to ingest and somewhat less painful than slitting one's own throat. Suicide at the death of a fiancé or husband, though not as mandatory as the Indian *suttee*, would gain the wife merit points in heaven. But a far larger proportion of suicides were motivated by a woman's need to gain revenge for wrongs inflicted, since the spirit of the suicide was believed to haunt and injure those who had been the cause. Both women and men committed, or at least attempted suicide with alarming frequency, because to ruin one's adversary one simply had to injure or kill oneself, preferably on the adversary's property. In some parts of China the person who caused the suicide might even be arrested and executed for the crime of murder. In any case, the perpetrator would be completely ruined and haunted forever by the victim's avenging ghost. For those who failed or were caught in the act, Leonora would have administered sulphate of copper, which made one Chinese so sick that he swore first, he would never taken opium again, and second, if he did, he would not send for foreign assistance![7]

Perhaps to help the cause of eradicating opium, the Victorian over-dramatization of the evil opium den was broadcast. On the proverbial dark and sinister night, an unsuspecting sailor is lured into a dimly lit, smoke-swirled room where menace lurks as surely as the Devil Himself. Induced to take a puff of smoke by a hand-wringing, slyly smiling Oriental, the sailor soon finds himself lost in a purgatory of addiction, raves like a lunatic, and offers his life savings and more for another puff.

In truth the "opium den" was more like a local pub where businessman and coolie alike went for an hour or so of relaxation. Wrote Somerset Maugham on his Chinese travels: "I was introduced into a neat enough room, brightly lit, divided into cubicles the raised floor of which, covered with clean matting, formed a convenient couch. In one an elderly gentleman ... was quietly reading a newspaper, with his long pipe by his side. In another two coolies were lying, with a pipe between them, which they alternately prepared and smoked. They were young men, of a hearty appearance, and they smiled at me in a friendly way. In a third four men squatted over a chess board, and a little further on a man was dandling a baby ... while the baby's mother ... watched him with a broad smile on her lips." Fiction, noted the famous author, was in this case stranger than fact.

But true addicts did exist. The worst were those wasted souls, the opium-eaters — not Thomas de Quincy's type* who swigged laudanum — but those so desperate that they ate the ash from the opium pipe. Tragically, Leonora would have weaned these addicts by using morphia, or morphine, in its stead. Although she and other physicians acted in good faith, their introduction of this drug created a huge new underground market for morphia, which was usually sold in lozenge form. The Western doctors' efforts exacerbated the problem tenfold, as morphia would prove far more lethal than the smoke produced by watered down poppy sap. In 1893, 15,000 ounces of hydrochlorate of morphia entered Shanghai. Much of it was prescribed to the Chinese by Western doctors.[8] Many Chinese women became even more addicted.

With the exception of Christian converts, the women Leonora treated had no rights at all in this patriarchal land. Few could read or write and, wrote one missionary, "While many of them have good minds, susceptible of taking even an advanced training ... to cook, wash and sew is looked upon as the sum of female duties." As girls were married, they were automatically transferred to the ownership of the husband's family, therefore education was waste of time and money. With no mental exercise and subject to much drudgery and abuse, they had little ambition and less hope. "In the Chinese language," wrote American Reverend R.H. Graves, "all that is weak, mean, little and debased is written with the radical for woman in it. Thus their estimate of the sex has become part of the very language itself."

One of Leonora's greatest heartbreaks must have been the treatment of China's little blind girls. With no chance of marrying them off, parents would sell them to street hags who trained them to "play the lute" and become, in the

*From de Quincy's book *Confessions of an English Opium-Eater.*

parlance of the times, singsong girls, or common prostitutes. "They are treated with great cruelty and are beaten if they do not return with something earned during the night," wrote Graves. "It is a common sight ... to see strings of six or eight of these girls, led by an old woman, going about the streets to ply their vocation." Their sunken eyes and sad thin faces were enough to excite the pity of the most unemotional. The Chinese themselves spoke of the blind girls' training houses as "little hells," so notorious were the cruelties practised on the inmates.[9] Though Chinese cities had provided charitable "blind asylums" for centuries, many officials turned their own blind eyes to the plight of these tragic, but sexually convenient, little slave girls.

As missionaries the world over knew, the key to enlightenment was education. Leonora's newest hospital was now a training ground for nurses, nurses' aides, and those who hoped to become doctors. It remains surprising that Li Hung-chang, himself extremely traditional within his family, would praise and encourage the uplift of Chinese women. It was, of course, Lady Li who sponsored Leonora's hospital, but it is unlikely she could have done so without his wholehearted approval. The Viceroy was a strange mixture, modern to the point of realizing the need for female physicians, and traditional enough to insist that his own daughter, in fact all female members of his family, remained cloistered in their palaces, tottering painfully around on their crippled "golden lilies."

Li had realized some years ago that continuance of the antiquated Chinese system of education was extremely dangerous for his beloved country. This system, for males only, had little to commend it in an increasingly modern world. As David Bonavia wrote in *The Chinese*, "On the traditional Chinese scale of priorities, education ranked only one notch below rice. To have a well-educated son was the pride and glory of any family that could afford the tuition fees." But in 19th-century China, education was nothing more than a lengthy process of learning calligraphy and memorizing classics, primarily literature and philosophy. Westerner and progressive Chinese alike agreed that China's largest mistakes lay in ignoring various hard sciences like mathematics and engineering skills, skills that Li knew could enable his country to resist increasing Western aggression.

Upon entrance to primary school — a major cause for celebration — each boy would be given a *shu ning*, or "book name" by which he would be known for the rest of his life. A typical schoolroom contained tables, benches, a teacher's chair, some ink stones, and a number of noisy young boys. The process involved tracing printed ideographs placed beneath very thin paper that were corrected here and there by the teacher. After writing the boys would shout their lessons at the top of their lungs to impress upon the teacher that they knew the subject. The monotony of memorizing went on for about two years, then, when the boys were familiar with a few thousand forms and sounds, the teacher would finally explain the meanings of the words. This system, stressing the Confucian values of filial piety, respect for elders, and a minutely detailed system of etiquette, had been for thousands of years the basis of education all over China, and had produced a veneration for letters unequalled in the world. Passing the final exams was also the only way, accident of birth aside, that a man could climb the ladder from peasant to Viceroy, or even, if the gods were willing, to Emperor.

School hours were long, lasting from sunrise until 10 am and from 11 am until early dusk. In villages and small towns, parents would pay the teacher from $3 to $6 a year and frequently offer small gifts of food.[10] Missionary educators, up against a frustrating obstacle that traditionally forbade social co-mingling among the sexes, frequently offered similar inducements, including accommodation. Other missionaries stipulated that for every two boys admitted to the school, the family would have to provide one girl student.

Not all missionaries — Leonora and Alex among them — were comfortable with the extreme emotional intimacy of evangelical education, feeling, perhaps, that the amount of sentiment expressed in revival meetings was just a bit too much to bear. Religious emotion, wrote one scholar, sometimes seemed to have substituted completely for content.[11] Maybe they were trying too hard, because even professionals like Leonora were disconcerted by the total lack of response shown by Chinese students. North American women who were used to speaking their minds and openly expressing emotion, felt stymied by the wall they encountered. Picture a gigantic Western schoolmistress attempting to instil "pep" into the tiny, feminine Chinese women and girls of the 19th century. Some tried rousing music and hymn-sings, others sports and organized outings. One actually wrote that her Chinese associates were learning better every year to be "informal and folksey." To children used to being surrounded with colour, noise, and an infinite variety of foods, missionary school surroundings were often deeply depressing.

One young girl of good family, but whose birthdate was considered inauspicious, was packed off to missionary school in Peking. To a nine year-old, this institute was a grim place indeed. Teachers with long noses and severe faces would have added to her terror. Fellow students were dispossessed paupers, which made her stand out even more than her youth. After six months, the little one had begged to be removed, as the food itself became insufferable: "every day the same old rice, corn muffins, also the unoiled old salty vegetables [probably tinned] which I can't eat." When her well-dressed mother arrived at the school, she found that better quality food could be obtained for a price. The money changed hands and the girl stayed put.

Although many missionaries admired Confucian ethics, they also felt alienated by a religion that hadn't any "life," and those who believed deeply in original sin faced a fairly large obstacle when faced with a population that believed in the merit principle.

Others like Leonora and Alex were more moderate in their views, and stuck to the original missionary principle of never interfering in a country's customs and politics. Not so some of the missionary society types at home who, in their comfortable London clubs, felt little but contempt for "the heathen." Leonora, who remained a strong but gentle soul, had married a shy and equally gentle mate. Perhaps her strength was rubbing off on him, because he began to take the side of the Chinese over stern, unbending edicts from home. With their more moderate viewpoints the couple had now won the trust and affection of the Chinese, whereas fundamentalists breathing fire and brimstone were routinely stoned, threatened, and sometimes killed.

Although the woman missionaries in Peking were also, for the most part, a moderate lot, there was still a distinct patronizing tone in their dealings with the Chinese. Annie Sears, who had now spent some years in China, reported the death of "dear old Chen Nai Nai, the school matron," as follows. "One woman came up and told me she found her crying because she had no way in which to pay me for my care of her. It was so touching ... to hear her beg the Lord to forgive her sins for my sake!" she wrote. "To look in *my face*, and not at her sins!" Annie Sears put her attitude in a nutshell when she continued "how sweet to her ears has been the 'Well done, good and faithful.'" Much to Miss Sears' delight, another, perhaps more suitable Mrs. Chen soon arrived in the "good and faithful's" stead. "She is 67, bright, intelligent, well-to-do, and clean," crowed Annie Sears. Intelligent Mrs. Chen was — and certainly not without wit. When studying the catechism and thinking herself "very stupid" she was told by Annie Sears to ask God to help her. The Chinese woman said "I have asked Him" but I guess He don't know. He has not got the news yet that I have come in here."

There is no hint of a patronizing attitude on the part of Leonora and her new husband, both of whom seemed to understand the social dilemmas that the Chinese converts faced. On July 25, 1894, a more confident, more mature Alex would write to his superior in London, "Dear Mr. Thompson: In your letter ... you state that the Board considered the punishment inflicted on Mr. Chang chin seng the theological tutor too lenient. ... Mr. Chang fell into the sin of bigamy simply from want of Christian courage to stand up against a common custom ... the Committee was extremely anxious while inflicting punishment to leave Mr. Chang a door of hope in the event of his future conduct showing that he was truly repentant. If he had been dismissed immediately I fear he would have been lost not only to the mission but to the Church. ... I should add that as soon as Mr. Chang was dismissed by the Committee he was deprived of Church membership by the native Church in Tientsin." Alex's petitions on behalf of Mr. Chang would continue for the next two years, and Mr. Chang would be reinstated.

As Li Hung-chang had predicted, the old Chinese system of education was now seriously eroding an empire that had been crumbling for centuries. Even the government's Educational Department was not free from bribery and corruption and this meant that those with a sufficient amount of money often found ways and means of purchasing their degrees — degrees that would ensure a comfortable government post for the rest of their lives. Li, who had risen from scholar to almost omnipotent Viceroy, saw the situation with his usual clear eyes and level head. As far back as 1881, he had complained: "The stupidity and confusion of our scholar officials, and the lack of men of ability in the court are really ridiculous."[12] If Westernized education could produce such forces as Britain, France and Germany, it was time for China to dispense with her stultified, often corrupt, educational system and concentrate more on technical advances.

Li had organized China's first "real" railway* and organized the North Sea Navy in 1881. In that same year China's first telegraph system appeared between Tientsin and Shanghai. By 1883, he had built ten warships, one christened *Li Shun De* — the same name as the Astor House Hotel, in which Li had a large interest. By 1894, this ill-fated vessel would play another part in Leonora's destiny. Five years later the hotel would play a similar part in her story.

Endnotes

1. *Woman's Foreign Missionary Society Eighteenth Annual Report*. Chicago: The Society, 1887, pp. 31-33.
2. Morrison, G.E. (Chinese). *An Australian in China*. Sydney, Australia: Angus and Robertson Pty. Ltd., 1972, p. 46.
3. Ibid., p. 191.
4. Ibid., p. 47.

*The British laid the very first railway in 1876 without permission. The Chinese tore it up.

5. Latourette, K.S. *A History of Christian Missions in China*. London: Society for Promoting Christian Knowledge, 1929, p. 458.
6. Morrison, *An Australian in China*, p. 45.
7. Ibid., p. 212.
8. Ibid., p. 49.
9. Graves, R.H. *Forty Years in China or China in Transition*. Baltimore, Maryland: R.H. Woodward Company, 1895, p. 110.
10. Bird, Isabella. *The Yangtze Valley and Beyond*. London: Virago Press Limited, 1985, p. 271
11. Hunter, Jane. *The Gospel of Gentility - American Women Missionaries in Turn-of-the-Century China*. New Haven: Yale University Press, 1984, p. 185.
12. Warner, Marina. *The Dragon Empress: Life and Times of Tz'u-hsi, 1835-1908, Empress Dowager of China*. London: Cardinal, 1974, p. 144

Chapter sixteen

The Japanese
1893–1895

"My country is hampered by traditions and customs ..."
— Li Hung-chang to Ito Hirobumi, 1895

Alex King had now become secretary of the London Missionary Society's Peking District Commission. Reports to London showed that over the years this shy Scottish vicar had learned how to work with both Chinese and home office alike. Leonora's hospitals were running smoothly with the help of Chinese money, and Alex's own business revolved around building more churches and schools.

Probably with Li Hung-chang's permission, Alex and his compatriots also took over a small temple and turned it into a Christian "service house." The temple, named *Hsiao Shen*, was called Charcoal Cross Temple by British soldiers. Then John Innocent, another missionary named John Shaw Burdon and Alex concentrated on building another church near Majiakou. These two churches had proven so popular that they could not hold all the foreigners, including soldiers, plus the burgeoning Christian convert population. A Danish vice-admiral named Steen Bille recorded that nearly all the foreigners in Tientsin took part in the construction of the next church, and found the scene quite moving. All in all, the Protestants built five churches in Tientsin. Three remain to this day.[1]

In 1891, Leonora and Alex took the long-awaited trip home, first to brother Eugene in Canada, and second to England, where they were issued huge tissue-thin passports, because Leonora intended to take some medical courses in Vienna. It was at this point that she learned to loathe England, specifically because its cold, damp climate wrought havoc with her health. From this time onward, she categorically refused to return to Alex's homeland, and it is likely she cut the visit short to return to China.

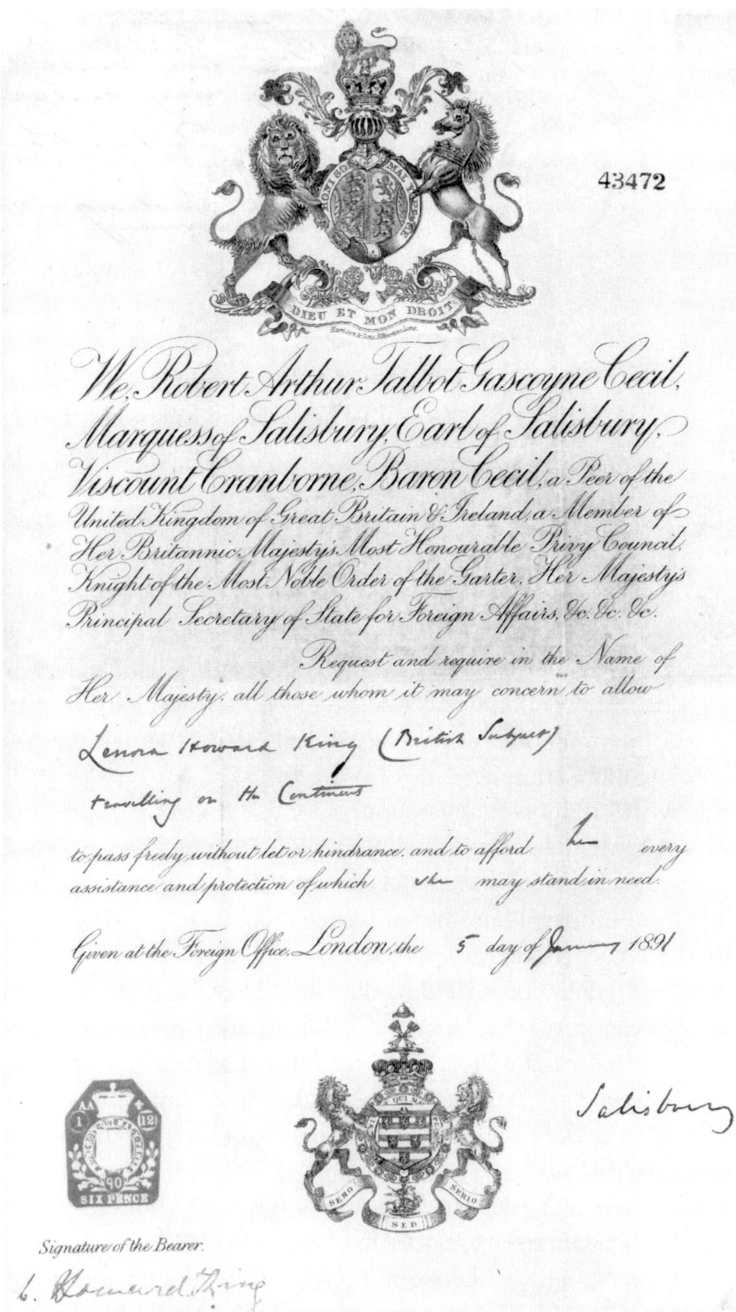

DIEU ET MON DROIT

43472

We, Robert Arthur Talbot Gascoyne Cecil, Marquess of Salisbury, Earl of Salisbury, Viscount Cranborne, Baron Cecil, a Peer of the United Kingdom of Great Britain & Ireland, a Member of Her Britannic Majesty's Most Honourable Privy Council, Knight of the Most Noble Order of the Garter, Her Majesty's Principal Secretary of State for Foreign Affairs, &c. &c. &c.

Request and require in the Name of Her Majesty, all those whom it may concern to allow

Leonora Howard King (British Subject)

travelling on the Continent

to pass freely without let or hindrance, and to afford her every assistance and protection of which she may stand in need.

Given at the Foreign Office, London, the 5 day of January 1891

SIX PENCE

SERO SED SERIO

Salisbury

Signature of the Bearer.

L. Howard King

Leonora's passport for "travelling on the continent"

A severe heat wave now crippled Chihli Province — heat, said the Chinese, such as had not been felt for 30 years. Owing to unusually heavy rains, tremendous damage was done to the missionary property, and Alex pressed the Home Office for more funding. Alex did, however, also keep London informed of Leonora's well-being. In 1893, it was not good. Perhaps owing to mosquito plagues that inevitably followed heavy rains — perhaps due to overwork in the sweltering weather, Leonora again fell ill. On August 5, Alex wrote that she had taken a bad turn, but was gradually, painfully, getting back on her feet.[2]

Leonora's frequent bouts with illness combined with her hard work had kept her reed-thin. She was now 42 years old. Her red-gold hair was dramatized with a broad streak of grey, and she had become a handsome, self-possessed woman. Her brisk, slender figure was by now a familiar sight throughout Tientsin, what with daily treks to her clinics and teaching hospital, or her personal calls at the private homes of wealthy Chinese. As befitted her profession, she dressed in sober colours, but often wore a feminine touch of white lace at her throat. Her luxuriant hair, always in the characteristic French twist, was usually adorned with one of many beautiful Chinese ornaments. Leonora had become a great lover of hats, which in those pre-Edwardian days, were often huge confections of tulle, feathers, or great silk cabbage roses.

Leonora's success now rested almost entirely on Chinese shoulders. It was a matter of "face" for anyone who could afford it to make contributions to her hospitals, in order that the poverty stricken may be treated. This adherence to the Confucian merit principle, while not as selfless as some Christians might have liked, remained a good source of income for many missionaries. And while letters to the missionary Home Offices invariably asked for extra funding from abroad, the Chinese themselves had entered into a neat give-and-take relationship with the long-nosed foreigners. It was now common knowledge that daughters could be saved from lives of slavery by being "sold" to missionaries. The missionary women were happy to pay a reasonable sum to save the little girls' souls. Those students who became true converts were used to spread The Word, and perhaps raise funds, in surrounding villages.

The work that Dr. Lucinda Coombs had started in 1872 and that Leonora had taken over in 1877 had blossomed into a bustling enterprise. By 1891, the North China Mission had 13 full-time woman workers, four physicians, two "on the field," three boarding schools with 172 pupils, three training schools for 48 Chinese Bible Women, one industrial school, 11 day-schools with 130 pupils, two hospitals, and three dispensaries.[3] Medical work was still centred in Tientsin rather than Peking — another of Leonora's legacies to the WFMS. There was a city clinic, held twice a week, a daily clinic at the hospital dispensary, ward treatment, and an extensive outpractice. The figure for the Isabella Fisher Hospital group alone was 11,167 patients for the fiscal year 1890–1891.

"Hospital patients have been unusually promising," said the report from the American missionary women. "Some have believed. Others have gone to their homes with a knowledge of the truth, which will bear fruit." Like other missionaries all over China, the women of Tientsin often faced incredible odds such as famine and flood, but their faith, under the circumstances, was nothing short of remarkable. "There is much in the past year's experience to prove that the practice of medicine among the women of North China from a purely professional point of view, is not inspiring;" wrote one Methodist, "but turn the missionary electric light full upon it, then it is that we forget the long rides through filth and wretchedness ... the weary struggle to understand and make ourselves understood in this tangled and entangling language, forget the weary days and sleepless nights spent in a hand-to-hand fight with poverty, filth, vermin, superstition and death, and thanking God, take courage and send the glad shout across the waters: 'The Lord's work prospers.' "[4]

In 1892, the Emperor issued an edict favourably mentioning missionary work and acknowledging the missionaries' "legal position" in his empire. The edict, granting full permission for Chinese to become Christians without in the least lessening their loyalty to their government, was placarded in the mission chapels of North China. This did not, wrote one WFMS member, mean that all opposition had been silenced, but some of the most serious obstacles were disappearing, and opportunities for aggressive work were never greater than at the present time. The doctors in Tientsin were busier than ever, but many echoed Leonora's earlier words to the WFMS Board back home. "We regret exceedingly *our* inability to do Evangelistic work with the medical. When the times comes that we can ourselves teach, as well as *heal*, and can carry the Gospel into every home...then, and not until then, shall we feel that we are fulfilling our whole mission."

In November 1891, the announcement of a local rebellion just outside the Great Wall, only a few miles from Tsun Hwa, itself fairly close to Tientsin, caused a great panic. The rebels' fury was, wrote the missionaries, specifically directed against foreigners and Christians. At first the local magistrate was much confused by the clamour of the people, and had advised the missionaries to leave at once for Tientsin, actually furnishing a conveyance and an escort for the journey. "News was received soon of the defeat of the rebels, when he [the magistrate] issued a proclamation, making provision for the protection of all mission property, so that when the missionaries returned, they found everything they had left behind safe and undisturbed." The local rebellion had, for a few months, lowered attendance at Leonora's hospital, as many women were afraid to venture out, particularly if they were caring for small children. But still "the work" continued, as she herself ventured into the streets and countryside, attending those who could not, or would not, come to the city.

Anti-foreign foment was still growing in outlying regions, because sometimes the missionaries just did not understand the severe strictures of Chinese etiquette. Much of the rage was directed toward Chinese converts — easier targets than the somewhat protected Westerners. Leonora's colleagues in Peking reported that in 1893, 20 young girls from Shantung, a 16-day journey from Peking, encountered great difficulty as they passed through various villages on their way to boarding school in Peking. The people of the villages took them to be "bad girls," as they were only accompanied by one male from the Christian college. Luckily one of the Christian helpers came to their rescue, locking them in a room and defending them against an angry mob of men. Officials in the villages refused to protect these young girls, because it was contrary to Chinese custom for them to travel in such a manner. After they reached Peking in safety, it was decided it would not be wise to send them home at the close of the school, and the unfortunate girls remained at school over the long summer vacation.

In Tientsin, Leonora's efforts were earning great dividends. Patients were remaining longer for treatment, which gave her the satisfaction of sending them home well, rather than temporarily patched up. An increasing number submitted to and sometimes even demanded surgical operations, because such action usually resulted in quick and satisfactory results. But still there was frustration when working for "the Cause." Although the missionaries attempted to explain the meaning of philanthropy to well-off Chinese ladies, there were few visible results. While being very generous in bestowing presents upon Leonora, they remained disinclined to give money to help the other missionaries buy medicines for the poor.

Back in 1889, Empress Dowager Tz'u-hsi had formally abdicated in favour of the Kuang-Hsu Emperor, who had reached the age of majority. The Emperor was slightly built and like many before him, in chronic ill-health. Two years before he ascended the throne he had been diagnosed with a lung condition of 12 years' standing, having already contacted bronchitis, emphysema, and perhaps tuberculosis. When the Emperor's father Prince Ch'un died in 1891, the young man found himself more and more reliant on his equally young concubines and his tutor Weng T'ung-ho, a 61 year-old practised statesman who had known him since he was a child. Weng described the technical advances and inventions of the West, and Kuang-hsu became fascinated with such items as clocks, which he bought by the dozen, then took apart and attempted to rebuild. The Emperor, sickly though he was, also plunged into astronomy, zoology, geology, physiology, law and political philosophy. It was rumoured, though not confirmed, that he was actually reading the New Testament. This may have had its grounds in the fact that Kuang-hsu began learning English with American missionary W.A.P. Martin, but he did not, in fact, make much headway.[5]

The year 1894 was to be one of great celebration, for the Empress Dowager would turn 60 years of age. She was planning a birthday party that would resound throughout the Empire, and in the process, leave a lot of officials painfully strapped for money. This must have worried Leonora and a number of other missionaries who depended on their generosity. All officials were expected to contribute 25 percent of their salaries to her birthday fund, and silks, robes, furs, jewels and delicacies of every sort would make their way through a poverty-stricken China to her opulent court.[6] Unfortunately for Tz'u-hsi, but fortunately for her officials, the party never took place. Korea, still turbulent after Sino-Japanese arrangements in 1885, became fraught with rebellion. In March 1894, the leading pro-Japanese reformer was lured to Shanghai and murdered, his corpse returned as a warning to sympathizers.

On July 23, the Japanese kidnapped the Korean queen and her children, and installed the 80-year-old father of the king as their puppet. British Major Hannekon commanded Li Hung-chang's ship *Kaoshing* and set sail for Korea. Having failed to force Hannekon and his Chinese troops to surrender, the Japanese cruiser *Naniwa* first fired a mine, which missed its mark. But after 30 minutes of steady bombardment the *Kaoshing* was sunk. The Japanese, reported Hannekon, shot at survivors in the water and killed 1,130 people. One hundred and seventy people, including the British commander, managed to make it to shore. Two days after that the puppet octogenarian on Korea's throne declared war on China.

On September 17, Hannekon took Li Hung-chang's warship, the *Li Shun*, to sea. (The "De" which means "morality" had been removed from the ship's name, as it could not be considered in terms of fighting with the enemy. A powerful Emperor was defeated in battle because he took morality as far as refusing to hurt wounded, young people and seniors on the battlefield.)[7] This time the ship managed to return, damaged but still triumphant, to the Taku Forts outside of Tientsin. The wounded and maimed from this ship and others flooded into Leonora's hospitals, and the city began to swell with refugees.

On October 3, Leonora's husband wrote from Tientsin, "Dear Mr. Thompson: ... I now hear definitely that the British Minister has required ladies and children to leave Peking so we expect all our Mission ladies here next week. The news of assaults on foreigners in the Capital was made too much of. Dr. Dudgeon was jostled because he resented some disrespectful language. ... As for Tientsin we have five gunboats in the river opposite the settlement — English, American, French, German and Russian ... the foreigners here (including the missionaries!) have been formed into an army — strictly for defensive purposes." The air, Alex continued, was full of rumours. "The respectable natives," he wrote, "are scared." Many of these "respectable natives" — those who could afford it — went south to escape the danger. Many more armed themselves to defend their property. "We quite expect the Japanese to make a vigorous attempt to enter Peking," Alex reported. "... local uprisings against the government may occur. ... All the mission [dwellings] will be outside the barricades — only the English settlement [where Leonora and Alex lived] and a small part of the French being considered defendable." The daily preaching, he added ironically, had little influence on people whose minds were full of war.[8]

The heavens, as well as the Japanese, saw fit to make life as hellish as possible. On October 18, Alex's supervisor W.H. Rees wrote that "the rains have been phenomenal. Hundreds of lives lost. The water was on all sides of our compound from 3 to 12 feet deep." On a more comic note, Rees and "Mack," or Dr. Mackenzie, had tied washtubs together to navigate around town. In the midst of this chaos, a number of missionary ladies arrived from Peking, against their wishes, to spend the winter. Leonora, on the other hand, might well have been overjoyed at this new influx of workers, for her hospitals remained flooded with wounded and dying Chinese soldiers, and sailors. At this time she closed her hospitals to women and children, concentrating, probably at Li Hung-chang's request, on saving as many military lives as possible.

Li struggled hopelessly to defend the vulnerable northeast entrance to his capital. The Japanese, armed to the teeth with Western weapons, drove him back across Korea to the Western border, then across the Liaotun peninsula on the Bay of Pechili, all the way to the Chinese citadel of Port Arthur. This fortress fell to the Japanese on November 21, 1894. Weihaiwei, another Western-style fortress across the Bay of Pechili, surrendered February 12, 1895. The admiral in charge of Li's navy committed suicide. His second-in-command, then the general in command of the forts, and another commanding officer, followed suit. Tz'u-hsi, thwarted from holding her huge birthday party, complained "Who would have anticipated that the dwarf men [the Japanese] would have dared to force us into hostilities?"[9]

By January 19, 1895, all was still quiet in Tientsin. "We do not expect any trouble now till the close of the war," wrote Alex. "Most of the batch of 300 wounded soldiers in the hospitals here have gone away [but] Mrs. King and Dr. Smith* have still a few soldiers in their hospitals." It is worthy of mention that Alex's concern for his Chinese deacon remained intact. Poor Mr. Chang, still evicted from the LMS church, was not neglected in all the troubles. A hasty note dashed off on January 30 mentioned that the "future of Mr. Chang had a very depressing effect on our Tientsin Church; and the war has been a very real hindrance." Sooner or later London would unbend.

Blame for the defeat by the Japanese was conveniently placed on the head of the 72 year-old Viceroy Li Hung-chang, who was summarily stripped of his titles but spared his life. Ironically it was the Japanese who brought Li back to prominence almost immediately. Rejecting the first peace envoys from China, they demanded a truly eminent representative in the ensuing negotiations. Li was now appointed ambassador and sailed for Shimonoseki, Japan. In victory, the Japanese demanded ownership of the Liaotung Peninsula, complete with Port Arthur, the Pescadores Islands and Formosa, concurrently under attack by their own fleets. But now a curious quirk of fate forced the Japanese to modify their demands. When Li Hung-chang arrived in Japan he was shot in the cheek by a fanatic. The bullet, it was said, just missed his eye. This near-assassination of such an eminent ambassador raised such an outcry from a previously silent Western community that the Japanese withdrew two of their original demands — one for more territory in Manchuria, and another for 300 million taels in silver.

Li Hung-chang signed the Treaty of Shimonoseki on April 17, 1895. In defeat he explained to the great Japanese statesman and reformer, Ito Hirobumi, "My country is hampered by traditions and customs; one can hardly do what one wants. China also has people who understand modern affairs; but there are too many provinces, with strong sectionalism, just like your country in the feudal period, when one was checked and hindered by others and had no full authority for anything."[10] Then using his philosophy of "play one barbarian to control another," he trusted Western nations to maintain a balance of power in China. On his own suggestion Russia, France and Germany 'requested' Japanese withdrawal from Liaotung. The Japanese did so, at the price of another 30 million taels.

Li in defeat was unpopular with both the court and the masses. In order to let the anger die down, Empress Dowager Tz'u-hsi whisked him to Russia as China's representative at the coronation of doomed Tsar Nicholas II. Li was either getting a bit old for intrigue or honestly trusted the Russians, for one year later a secret treaty would bind these two great countries to defend each other

*Smith would have taken over Kenneth Mackenzie's hospital after Mackenzie retired.

against Japan. China, through Li, actually granted Russia the right to extend the Trans-Siberian railway across Manchuria to the sea, and to transport troops and military supplies not only in times of war with Japan, but in times of peace. Li was accused of taking bribes from the Russians, but Count Witte, that country's negotiator, denied this calumny in his own memoirs.

On July 23, 1895, Alex and Leonora travelled to Nanking. Li Hung-chang had asked Leonora to render some medical service to his daughter, who had gone south during the war. "His Excellency himself suggested I should accompany Mrs. King ... I can easily get away for a month," pleaded Alex. "The Viceroy," he added hastily, "pays all expenses." Even in disgrace with the Ch'ing court, Li Hung-chang would do a lot more than that.

Shortly after the end of the war, British Major Hannekon was promoted to the rank of general and asked by the Emperor to take charge of the Imperial Chinese Army. Very shortly after that Mrs. Leonora Howard King, MD, was awarded the Imperial Order of the Double Dragon.

Endnotes

1. Liu Jiantang and Tian Yutang, eds. *Astor Hotel Sightseeing Over a Century*. Tianjin, People's Republic of China: Tianjin People's Publishing House, 1993, pp. 333-334.
2. Council for World Missionary Archives, Day Missions Library, Yale University. London Missionary Society Records. Box H-2139, 8. 1893.
3. *Woman's Foreign Missionary Society 23rd Annual Report*. 1892, pp. 48-50.
4. *Woman's Foreign Missionary Society Annual Report*. 1891, pp. 36-39.
5. Warner, Marina. *The Dragon Empress: Life and Times of Tz'u-hsi, 1835-1908, Empress Dowager of China*. London: Cardinal, 1974, pp. 156-157.
6. Ibid., p. 178.
7. Liu Jiantang and Tian Yutang, eds., *Astor Hotel Sightseeing Over a Century*, p. 259.
8. Council for World Missionary Archives, Day Missions Library, Yale University. London Missionary Society Records. Box H-1239. 1895.
9. Warner, *The Dragon Empress*, p. 180.
10. Ibid., p. 148.

Chapter seventeen

Winds of war
1896–1899

Ye have not chosen me, but I have chosen you.
— John 15:16

In 1896, there were 750 Roman Catholic priests with half a million converts, and 1,300 Protestant missionaries with a somewhat more disappointing 55,000 new Christians.[1] Dr. Sun Yat-sen, a missionary-trained physician who would become the father of China's revolution, was detained in the Chinese Legation in England. Dr. Leonora Howard King of Farmersville, Ontario, became the first Western woman to be made a mandarin. She was 44 years old.

The Empress Dowager may have presided at the ceremony at the Forbidden City in Peking. As no outsider was allowed to gaze upon Tz'u-hsi's face, Li Hung-chang would have conferred the honour upon a kneeling Leonora. The court itself would have been filled with crown princes, richly dressed eunuchs, and perhaps both the British and American ambassadors. The royal ladies, who were not at this time supposed to be seen by foreigners, would watch from another court. After having the order conferred, Leonora would probably retire to the company of these ladies.

The Imperial Chinese Order of the Double Dragon, which originated in 1882, had a hierarchy as complex and endless as the Empress Dowager's wardrobe. The Order was divided in the first place into five classes, each of which was subdivided, with eleven grades in all. The highest class had a first division destined for sovereigns, a second for princes and a third for the hereditary nobility. The second-class order, which Leonora may have received, had a first division for ambassadors, a second for lesser diplomats, a third for diplomatic officials, and so on. Leonora's Order was in the shape of a Celtic cross, with two dragons roaring in the centre. In the upper part a star in green and blue was adorned with a glowing ruby.[2]

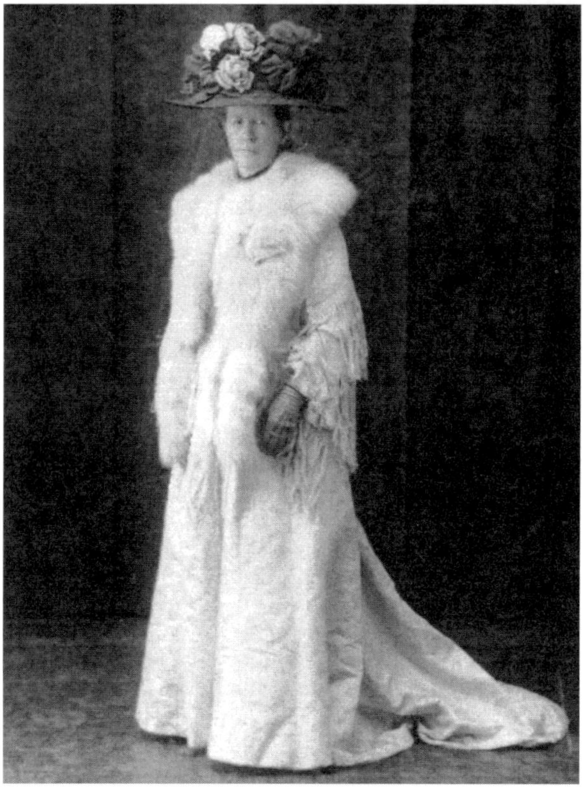

Off to the palace

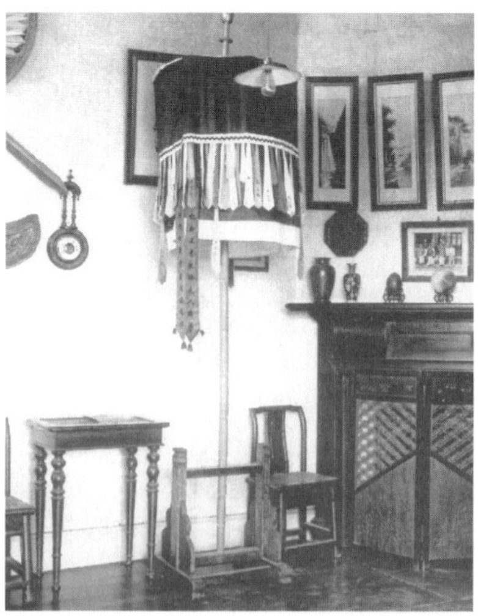

The ceremonial umbrella

By being awarded this high honour, Leonora joined the ranks of such revered Westerners as General "Chinese" Gordon, who had actually become a first-rank mandarin in 1863 in recognition of his brilliant campaign against the Taiping rebels. Gordon was the only person other than the Emperor and Empress allowed to wear the Imperial yellow. Leonora was, however, now allowed to wear ermine, the fur reserved for Chinese royalty. With her rich ermine coat, lined with exquisite red Chinese silk, she made a formidable figure as she appeared at more and more public functions. As a mandarin, Leonora was also given an umbrella of honour, a tall circular device on a bamboo pole that announced the passage of people of importance. It is unlikely that she would have used the umbrella, perhaps with the exception of visits to the homes of Chinese royalty, where these trappings would now be expected. Leonora would also be one of the few missionaries to be embraced by the diplomatic community, most of whom still looked down on servants of God as somehow too dowdy for their enchanted inner circles.

Dowdy, Leonora decidedly was not. A picture taken about this time shows a very different doctor — an elegant figure clad in heavy pale silk with a train, rich white arctic fox furs, an enormous hat crowned with silken roses, and fine leather gloves. With silver and turquoise jewellery adorning her wrists and ears, she is fit to be presented at any diplomatic function or indeed, at any court in Europe. Had she, in fact, been in Europe, the Order would have been analogous to being given the title of Lady Howard King.

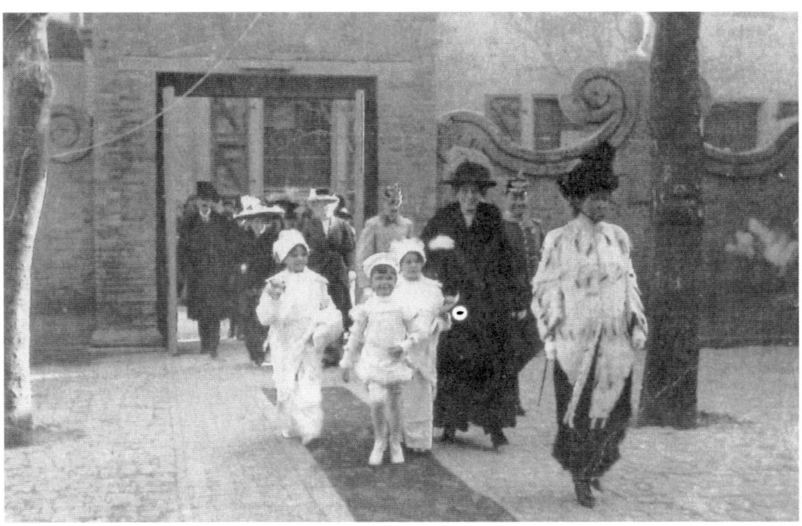

Leonora in Mandarin's ermine

Her mentor, His Excellency Li Hung-chang, returned home from Russia and a subsequent world tour, including a stop in Canada, in the winter of 1896. A letter from missionary Mrs. W.E. Smith, dated R.M.S. *Empress of China*, September 14, read:

> "To say the trip has been interesting is expressing it very mildly. We have on board a cosmopolitan company — pleasure seekers and invalids. French nobility represented, English aristocracy, and his Excellency Li Hung Chang and party, certainly *not least*. We have had the pleasure of having an interview with the latter to-day. It was very, very interesting. ... A Chinese doctor (educated in the hospital in Peking, [sic] established by Lady Li after her cure by Dr. Howard) acted in that capacity for us. His excellency was very interested in the work; enquired if hospitals had been rebuilt, how many we had there, how many schools, how many missionaries, how many years experience Dr. Smith had had, if I, too, understood medicine; regretted that I did not, as Chinese ladies would not be benefited by gentlemen doctors. Enquired very minutely how many of those who were expelled at the time of riots had returned to Canada, if any were still in China, if any had

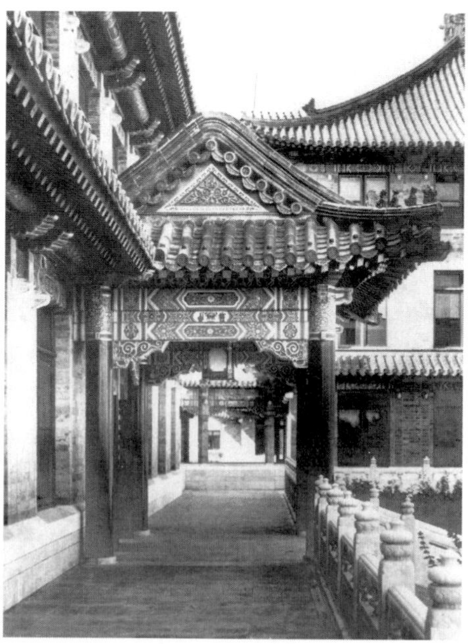

"Rockefeller" Hospital in Peking

> returned to Chen-tu, commended us for our courage, was glad we were going, hoped we would be very successful in medical work, and thus win the love and confidence of the people; if we could successfully treat disease he felt sure no such riots would re-occur. In bidding us good-bye His Excellency said, 'My reception in England and Canada has been so cordial that it is with pleasure I receive an Englishman or Canadian. I shall watch your career with interest, and if ever I can be of any help ... shall gladly do so.'
>
> "This *king among men* is seventy-four years old, yet his eye is bright and his countenance brightens as he speaks of the good to be done his people. ... Yesterday two lady missionaries from Toronto interviewed him, and in his farewell he said, "I am almost persuaded of the truth of the Gospel." ... His son, Lord Li Chang Hong, is also of the party, and very intelligent. Mr. Li Chung's [sic] son is the most studious man on board. ... He may be seen for hours each day reading. He says he has read the Bible, Darwin, Locke, and is willing to receive the Gospel if he could understand. He can understand Confucius; he told them to curb their passions and live pure lives. He made no pretensions to be other than a great prophet. Jesus Christ he cannot understand. He was a fool — he claims to be the Son of God. He asked what more he must to do become a Christian. Admitted he had gone no further than his reason led him, but could not quite see how he could believe on [in] the Lord Jesus Christ when he claimed such preposterous things."[3]

During Li's absence, Russia, France, England and Germany outdid each other in attempts to lend money to China, which was struggling to pay Japan's "indemnity" and to repair and retrench. Eventually China borrowed from all four, pledging customs revenue, and transit and salt taxes as security. In November the German Kaiser had been informed that "the Minister at Peking should be instructed to keep his eyes open for an event suitable as a cause for advance." In 1897, some Chinese bandits robbed a village in Shantung, burning the houses and murdering the inhabitants. Among the victims were two German missionaries. The Kaiser roared "Plentiful atonement ... must be secured by energetic action of the fleet. The squadron must instantly proceed to Kiaochow, seize the port there, and threaten with severest repression unless the Chinese government instantly agree to a high compensation in gold as well as a really effective pursuit and punishment of the criminals. I am fully determined to abandon, henceforth, the over-cautious policy which had been regarded by the Chinese as a weakness, and to show ... with full power and — if necessary — with brutal ruthlessness that the German Emperor cannot be made sport of and that it is bad to have him as an enemy."

The German Kaiser's obsession with the "Yellow Peril" inspired him to encourage the new Tsar, Nicholas II, to occupy himself with Far Eastern ambitions. In 1895, he had commissioned the German artist, H. Knackfuss, to create a picture showing (as he described it) "the Powers of Europe represented by their respective Genii called together by the Archangel Michael, sent from Heaven, to unite in resisting the inroads of Buddhism, heathenism, and barbarism, for the defence of the Cross," and he presented the first copy to the Tsar. Germany's immediate aim, however, was to challenge the empires of the British and French. Although Germany's commerce in China was second only to the British, she had no commercial bases like Hong Kong, no coaling station, no docking and repair facilities, and no fortified naval base.

In 1897, Kaiser Wilhelm wrote to Chancellor von Bulow in China: "Thousands of German Christians will breathe more easily when they know that the German Emperor's ships are near; hundreds of German traders will revel in the knowledge that the German Empire has at last secured a firm footing ... hundreds of thousands of Chinese will quiver when they feel the iron fist of Germany heavy on their necks. ... "[4] Apart from their fear of German intervention, the Russians were constrained by their treaties to support Chinese resistance to Wilhelm — and for a while they did so. Then the Russians pulled a *volte-face*, withdrawing their support for China. In 1898, the Tsungli Yamen, or Foreign Office, signed an agreement for the lease of Kiaochow.Kiaochow and a radius of 50 kilometres was subsequently leased to Germany for 99 years.

Then Russian warships sailed into Port Arthur and announced that they had come to stay. Count Witte did, this time, admit that he had paid Li Hung-chang and a Western colleague — probably Detring — 500,000 taels to expedite the matter. By March 1898, Port Arthur and nearby Talienwan were "leased" to Russia for 25 years, with all mining and railway rights for almost 100 kilometres around. England, represented by an inexperienced ambassador, Sir Claude Macdonald, joined the fray, demanding that since the balance of power in Pechili Gulf had been disrupted, Britain should take over Weihaiwei as soon as the Japanese indemnity had been paid and the town cleared. He also wanted an increase in land at Kowloon, just across the bay from British "leased" Hong Kong. France, not to be left in the lurch, used antimissionary riots in Canton to demand a 99-year lease on Kwangchowan, south of Hong Kong. The superpowers, now back to wining and dining each other, carved out spheres of influence, with the entire Yangtze basin from Szechuan to Kiangsu being British, southern Canton and Southern Yunnan French, a belt from Kansu through Sensi, Shansi, Hunan and Shantung German, and Manchuria and Chihli Province, home to Leonora and Alex King, being Russian. The Americans, staying clear of outright seizure, secured equal rights and opportunities for all nations, including the United States, in all leased areas.

Russian occupation or no, Leonora's medical work now began to get back on track. There had been a serious smallpox outbreak in Tsun Hwa, close to Tientsin, but it was now under control. Because country women were more receptive to Christianity than those from the city, field work was still an important part of her life. Travelling with Chinese Bible women in tow, Leonora might visit up to eight villages a day. The tiny women with sickly babies, the pale stoic little girls living with the pain of their bound feet, the ancient filthy beggar women always brought back the real China with a bump. No amount of cloistered living in the foreign concessions could ever diminish Leonora's tenderness toward the diseased and the destitute. The wonder was that any of the very poor had survived the war and floods at all, as food had become so scarce and expensive, but the return to peace and plenty of food for a few weeks made a wonderful change in the appearance of these women and children. A number of missionaries reopened their schools and hospitals, "though it was almost vacation time." This was done so that "the girls nearby might have *food*," wrote one missionary, "which was so scarce in their own homes, that they were *suffering*."[5]

Leonora, with support from the Chinese aristocracy, remained almost unique among the missionaries in refusing to charge for her work. Former colleagues in the WFMS now reported freely that it was becoming quite common for some Chinese families to secure medical services by the year,[6] and there did not seem to be any objection to this practice.

One of her most difficult and trying duties was to inform a patient and her relatives that even if they were willing to pay, nothing could be done to cure a particular disease. It was all the more tragic when the patient had been brought at much financial sacrifice, over many days' journey, buoyed with the hope of recovery. So many Chinese suffered from blindness, either through cataracts, which were treatable, through trachoma, which was more difficult to deal with, or, in the case of one poor soul, having quicklime rubbed into her eyes as a punishment for some transgression. The worst part of being blind in China was that one became despised, cast out from the family, and destined to spend the rest of one's life roaming the streets and begging for enough to eat.

Although Leonora spoke fluent Chinese, another source of great anxiety was an utter disregard by both patient and relatives of the explicit instructions she gave regarding medication. The doctor might give sufficient medicine for eight doses, to be taken every four hours, with strict warnings about the dangers of overdose. The next day she would hear that, owing to the severity of the pain, the patient had pleaded for the medicine and taken the whole bottle in the middle of the night. Similarly, after she had performed a successful cataract operation, friends might come to visit the patient, curious to inspect the eye or eyes. Contrary to imperative orders not to touch the bandages, the eyes would be uncovered for inspection, usually amid a cloud of smoke. Each friend who wanted to inspect the eyes would probably use dirty fingers to keep the eyelids open. This was often followed by infection, which resulted in total loss of sight. In all such cases the answer was "The patient wanted it," or "the friends wanted to see." To a Chinese mind, wrote one frustrated doctor, "that was reason enough for anything."

At this time, Leonora's and other missionary hospitals were said to be of the latest and most approved European type. Lighting, ventilation, general sanitation, arrangement and organization, and using *Ningpo* varnish, or lacquer, produced a very hard finish on the floors. A weekly rub with kerosene greatly aided sanitation.

But suicide was still rampant among Chinese women. These days, apart from taking overdoses of opium, a frequent mode of taking one's life was ingesting the heads of matches, which produced an agonizing death from phosphorus poisoning. Gold leaf, lead or magnesium chloride were also common, as was jumping down wells or into rivers. Women frequently cut their throats or stabbed themselves in the abdomen. Their lives were still little more than slavery. Something had to be done.

On June 11, 1898, Emperor Kuang-hsu announced the "Hundred Days of Reform Movement" in an effort to free China of debts to the foreigners and regain the land being snatched from under his very nose. The announcement, drafted by tutor Weng, read in part: "There must be a careful investigation of every branch of European learning, appropriate to existing needs, so that there may be an end to existing fallacies and that by zeal, efficiency may be attained." The young and delicate Emperor hastened to note that Empress Dowager Tz'u-hsi was responsible for all the new measures. Tz'u-hsi, fearing overthrow, banished tutor Weng and settled the all-important vice-royalty of Chihli Province upon her trusted adviser and cousin Jung-lu, who had been banished to the provinces seven years ago.

But the Emperor's educational reforms took hold: along with missionary W.A.P. Martin, who had been teaching him English, Kuang-hsu now established the fabled University of Peking. Manchus, those of the ruling classes, were urged to travel abroad; provincial schools taught skills such as the preparation of tea and silk; inventors and writers were encouraged by the introduction of patents and copyrights, and "unofficial" temples and shrines were ordered, somewhat like Leonora's first "temple-hospital," to become village schools. Finally, and probably to much rejoicing across the nation, the "eight-legged essay," the bedrock of the antiquated examination system, was temporarily abolished.

Kuang-hsu was not finished. Following Li Hung-chang's lead in Westernizing Chihli Province, the Emperor ordered officials to encourage and assist the hitherto-despised merchant class. He set up the Bureau of Control of Mines and Railways, and allowed fellow Manchus to take up professions. The badly trained Manchu Bannermen were to adopt Western drill, and soldiers to pass tests. Journalists were told to write on political matters, a reform of the law-courts was promised, and on August 24, 1898, the Emperor announced that on October 19, he and the Empress Dowager would actually travel, by train, in full view of the populace, to Tientsin. But on September 17, Kuang-hsu made a grave error. He dismissed Leonora's protector Li Hung-chang from the office where the highest decisions were made — the Tsungli Yamen.

Empress Dowager Tz'u-hsi was furious, but strangely she refused to reinstate Li and others who had been "fired." It would eventually take rumours of her overthrow to make her take action. These were conveniently provided by those loyal to the status quo. On September 22, the Emperor Kuang-hsu was "imprisoned" in the *Ying T'ai*, or Ocean Terrace, a paradise of a prison, with a drawbridge being the only exit. All the Emperor's personal eunuchs were changed, and word had it that 14 had been executed at the Empress Dowager's command. The favourite Pearl Concubine was arrested and confined to her rooms, but Empress Lung-yu, Tz'u-hsi's niece, was allowed to live with the Emperor. Tz'u-hsi issued on behalf of the Emperor, what amounted to an abdication, saying: "From this day forth her Majesty will transact the business of the government in the Side Hall of the Palace, and on the day after tomorrow we ourselves at the head of our Princes and Ministers shall perform obeisance before her."

Endnotes

1. Purcell, Victor. *The Boxer Uprising*. Cambridge: Cambridge University Press, 1963, p. 75.
2. In 1911, the badge was altered to a five-pointed star with blunt, widening points and with a central medallion bearing the double dragon. The star of the Grand Cross is eight-pointed and rayed, and the centre held a coral bead, ruby or sapphire. The ribbon of the higher grades is dark red and fringed.
3. Howard Family Collection. *The Missionary Outlook* (1896), p. 182.
4. Purcell, *The Boxer Uprising*, pp. 90-92.
5. *Woman's Annual Conference of the Methodist Episcopal Church, North China*. 1895, pp. 43-44.
6. *Woman's Foreign Missionary Society, North China Mission Annual Report*. 1894, p. 44.

Chapter eighteen

The Boxers
1899

"It sounded as if madness itself were let loose ..."
— Sarah Pike Conger

The Society of Righteous Harmonious Fists, or I Ho Chuan, had been known by many names. Some say they began as the Plum Blossom Fists, or perhaps the Eight Diagram Sect, or the Red Fist Society. The name Boxers was coined by two missionaries who frequently wrote for the *North China Daily News*. Back in 1895, these missionaries had noticed various youth-gangs exhibiting some curious behaviour. A teenager would fall to his knees within a circle of cohorts, and begin to chant in high-pitched wails. Drawing mystic signs in the dirt, he worked himself into a frenzy, eyes rolling back until only the whites were visible. Achieving an ecstatic, trance-like state, the youth would rise and begin ritualistic "shadow-boxing" exercises. "Uphold the Great Pure Dynasty and Exterminate the Barbarian!" the gangs would shriek.

Missionaries who had witnessed previous anti-foreign riots went about their daily work with outward serenity. No matter what they felt privately, any Old China Hand knew that just one expression of fear was enough to set off a bloody conflagration of east against west. It would, in fact, take almost two years before formal reports of the Boxers began to filter back to London.

In 1897, Alex's former supervisor William Rees wrote from the Chi Chou Medical Centre that the countryside was definitely in a state of unrest. Stories about recent kidnapping troubles in Tientsin had reached his district, he said, and as usual, "they have been greatly distorted and exaggerated." Anonymous placards had been posted up all over the region, instructing the people "to beware of us and to resort to lawlessness ... we should be buried alive ... and no official would hinder any persons doing such a thing."[1]

In Tientsin, Leonora faced a daily dilemma of convincing her patients to stay in hospital for treatment, rather than avoid the foreign magic medicine. Young girls in particular were a constant worry. They were often brought in half-conscious from ugly infections in their tiny bound feet. If gangrene had not yet set in, Leonora could at least supply some clean foot-bandages, a bit of sulfa and because she loved children so much, some good old-fashioned kindness. If gangrene had set in, the feet, or legs, would have to be amputated.

Explanations to patients who were nervous of the foreigners must have begun to sound like a broken record, so often was it necessary to calm the fears of the superstitious. As described previously, in 1870, some Roman Catholic nuns in Tientsin were wrongly accused of buying children, then murdering them in order to practise sorcery. It was true that the nuns, who ran an orphanage, had sometimes paid a few cash to save some pitiful child from slavery, and it was true that some of the children were so sick on arrival that they died soon afterward. The little graves on the orphanage grounds and the predictable jars of preserved cherries, presented as the eyes of the children, had provided enough evidence for a mob to slaughter every one of the nuns. The infamous "Tientsin massacre" stories — stories of Westerners killing children for purposes of magic — were making their rounds again.

That winter, flood and famine returned to Chihli province with a vengeance. More than 3,500 kilometres of precious wheat and cabbage were submerged in the malevolent waters of the Yellow River. Entire villages simply disappeared. At one point 150,000 people were squatting on broken dykes just inches above the swirling waters, silently watching the bloated bodies of dogs, cows, pigs and humans float by on the relentless current. Those who survived foraged for tree-bark and leaves to fill their distended bellies. When the waters receded and the sun dried the earth, plagues of locusts, believed to be sent by the spirit world, devoured what was left of the crops. Someone had to take the blame.

The arrogant foreigners neatly filled at least part of the bill. Always simmering close to the surface, anti-foreign bubbles of sentiment began to appear when Germans, occupying Kiaochow (Confucius' birthplace), the British in Weihaiwei, and the Russians in Liaotung decided that as leaseholders, they were entitled to the Chinese taxes gathered in those areas. The bubbles broke inexorably, one by one. In 1898, an English missionary was murdered in Kweichow. At about the same time, a French priest was tortured to death in Hupeh.

Paradoxically, Leonora's Western medicine was now needed even more desperately, as thousands of starving refugees poured into the cities in search of food and medicines. An appalling outbreak of typhoid followed the floods. Malaria, ever present in swampy Tientsin, felled hundreds more. Families of the dying clamoured to be allowed into the Western hospitals to accompany their relatives' departed souls on the road to immortality. Some were admitted. Most were turned away for fear of further infection.

Leonora also had her hands full with smallpox cases. "Though smallpox, like the poor, we have always with us," wrote WFMS colleague Dr. Iva Miller, "this winter it has been unusually virulent. ... One of us vaccinated sixteen children in one day." There was still room for humour on the wards, though. "One of the clean intelligent families, (there are many such in Tientsin), came in a flock to the doctor's study," she related. "They made such a cunning picture, the six of them ... grouped round the open fire drying their vaccinations, that, considering the fact that vaccination in the Chinese language is, 'Planting the flower,' the member of our household, who called another to see the doctor's flower garden, may be forgiven the sin of punning!"

Smallpox attacked Chinese and foreigner alike, though the latter were far more likely to die from the unfamiliar virus. Sarah Pike Conger, wife of the American ambassador, wrote at Thanksgiving: "There was one cloud that cast its shadow over this bright day. Our marines had gathered ... to join in our thanksgiving; the services had not yet opened when it was quietly whispered to Mr. Conger that one of the marines had smallpox. ... Mr. Conger thinking it best to tell those with us, made the announcement. Almost as with one voice the missionaries exclaimed "You cannot frighten us in that way; we come in contact with smallpox nearly every day of our lives." Sadly, the marine died in December.

For the moment, the Chinese populace still seemed divided on the issue of who to blame for the series of misfortunes. The Imperial family had, as usual, offered financial aid to the flood victims, but very little of it filtered down through the grasping hands of officialdom. In 1899, Canadian doctor James Frazer Smith reported "many violent and bloody encounters took place between the officials and these famished hordes. " Near the missionary stations at Changte, said Frazer Smith, about 100 hungry peasants took refuge in a temple. Chinese soldiers set the temple on fire and all hundred were burned to death, "as any who tried to escape were driven back into the burning building."[2]

In January 1899, the Empress Dowager decreed that all viceroys, governors and tartar-generals should from now on deal with foreign matters locally. In the same decree, she made the enormous error of giving missionaries equivalent rank with Chinese officials. This meant that the trappings already assumed by

Roman Catholic bishops — the mandarin's button, a retinue of chair-bearers and outriders, the umbrella of honour and the firing of a cannon on arrival or departure — were now granted them as a right, not a privilege, as had been won by Leonora. Tz'u-hsi may have hoped to control the Christians through the process of absorption, even as her own Manchu peoples had been absorbed into the mainstream Confucian culture over the centuries. Even though the Roman Catholics were the only Western religious group to accept such dangerous honours, justifiable outrage toward these arrogant foreigners erupted among even the most moderate Chinese.[3]

In April, Wu T'ing-fang, the Chinese minister to the United States, attempted to explain the anti-foreign sentiment by asking the American Academy of Political and Social Science to imagine that the Chinese had sent Confucian missionaries to America, established themselves in major cities, built temples, held public meetings, opened schools, and gathered round them a mass of converts. "If they were to begin ... by making vehement attacks on the doctrines of Christianity, denouncing the cherished institutions of the country, or going out of their way to ridicule the fashions of the day, perhaps giving a learned discourse on the evil effects of corsets ... it is most likely they would be pelted with stones, dirt and rotten eggs for their pains."[4] No one in China, at least, seemed to take any notice of his warnings.

The Italians, feeling left out of the race for Chinese concessions, now demanded the lease of San-men Bay in Checkiang. The British supported this claim by quietly placing a few gunboats off the coast. The Empress Dowager flatly refused to consider this latest insult, and summoned hundreds of Chinese troops to Peking. Secret decrees were issued stating that if the foreigners attacked, this time China would fight.

In October 1899, the Peking diplomatic corps, feeling they needed some protection, asked that 100 Allied troops be sent from Tientsin. At the end of the month, Imperial troops attacked a British diplomat and began to hover close to the legation quarter. Sir Claude MacDonald, the British minister (high commissioner), demanded that the troops withdraw immediately. Tz'u-hsi reluctantly complied.

The Empress Dowager's earlier edict had backfired in more ways than one. On November 11 she wrote:

> "Various powers cast upon us looks of tiger-like voracity, hustling each other ... to be the first to seize upon our innermost territories. They think that China, having neither money nor troops, would never venture to go to war ... whenever these high officials [the viceroys and governors] have had on their

> hands cases of international dispute, all their actions seem to be guided by the belief in their breasts that such cases would eventually be 'amicably arranged.'...when matters do come to a crisis, they, of course, find themselves utterly unprepared to resist any hostile aggression on the part of the foreigners ... we now find it incumbent upon ourselves to censure such conduct in the most severe terms." [5]

Curiously, at the same time Tz'u-hsi continued to court the foreign diplomats. On December 13, for her 64th birthday, she invited the senior legation ladies to tea. At 10 am a mounted Chinese escort went to each legation to escort the ladies to the British Legation, because Lady MacDonald was dean of the diplomatic wives, having been in China the longest. The women formed quite a procession, with 12 sedan chairs and 60 bearers. "We stood according to rank (longest time in Peking)," wrote American Sarah Conger, "and bowed." This was more than most male Westerners did in the presence of their imperial majesties, and it is likely that the Empress Dowager was pleased by this courtesy.

The ladies were introduced to the Emperor and Empress Dowager by Prince Ch'ing, then "She offered both her hands and we stepped forward to her. With a few words of greeting, Her Majesty clasped our hands in hers, and placed on the finger of each lady a heavy, chased gold ring, set with a large pearl." After luncheon with Prince and Princess Ch'ing and five other princesses, the diplomatic wives took tea in another room, then invited back to the banquet-hall. "To our surprise, there on a yellow throne-chair, sat Her Majesty. ... She was bright and happy and her face glowed with good will. There was no trace of

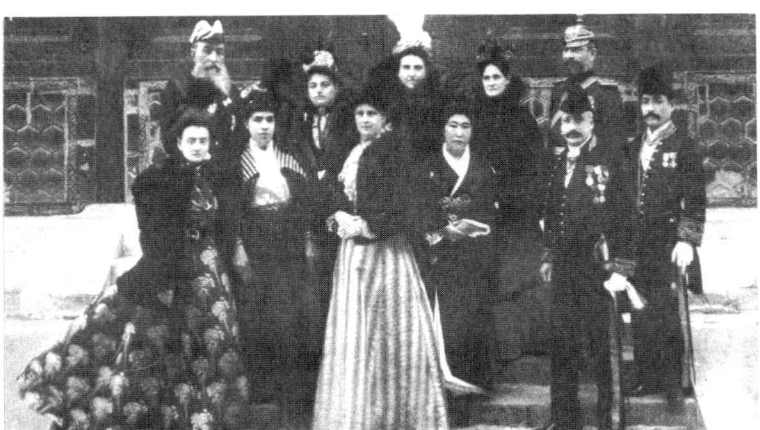

Ladies and gentlemen of the legations

cruelty to be seen. ... She extended both hands toward each lady, then, touching herself, said with much enthusiastic earnestness, 'One family; all one family.' "

After viewing a play, they were once more in Tz'u-hsi's presence. The Empress Dowager tipped each lady's cup of tea to her own lips, took a sip, then lifted the cup, on the other side, to their lips, again saying "One family, all one family." She presented more beautiful gifts, and the ladies returned home, enthralled.[6]

At the end of the month the foreign elite greeted the new century with grand style: white tie joined glittering ballgown in toasting the centenary with the best champagne. While the diplomats and the less-rigid missionaries danced that New Year's Eve, the Boxers tortured a young English missionary named Brooks, finally giving him the mercy of death. The murderers were arrested and executed within a few days, and the Tsungli Yamen, the Bureau of Foreign Affairs,* expressed formal regrets. This would be the last time it followed normal diplomatic procedure.[7]

Tientsin, that bastion of Westernization, was awash with rumour. Leonora's hospitals, her heart and her soul, became emptier as the days went by. In the past months, she had survived yet another savage attack of malaria that left her frail and feverish. During her enforced absence at her country home in Peitaiho, even the most educated houses had closed their heavy doors to the foreigners. With little to do in his empty church, Alex, as district secretary, kept in constant touch with missionary stations in the interior.

The situation there was quite the opposite from the ghost town that Tientsin had become. Many inland missionaries worked day and night to save the lives of, or more sadly, to bury the "Secondary Devils" (Chinese Christians) who had been attacked and tortured by the Boxers. Some of the viceroys in other provinces offered to protect the Westerners. The Chinese converts could fend for themselves.

On January 11, 1900, the Empress Dowager issued an edict that in essence would give the Boxers free reign. It stated, in part, that:

> "Of late in all the Provinces brigandage has daily become more prevalent, and missionary cases [attacks] have recurred. ... Most critics point to seditious societies as the cause, and ask for rigorous suppression ... but reflection shows that societies are of different kinds. When worthless vagabonds form them-

*A "yamen" was a governor's office, both physically and officially. The Tsungli Yamen was the highest office in the land, made up of Princes and Viceroys. Li Hung-chang was a member of the Tsungli Yamen.

> selves into bands ... and ... create disturbances, the law can show absolutely no leniency. ... On the other hand when peaceful and law-abiding people practise their skill in mechanised arts for the preservation of themselves and their families, or when they combine ... for the mutual protection of the rural population, this is in accord with the public-spirited principle of 'keeping mutual watch and giving mutual help.' "

Two days prior to the Empress's pronouncement, missionaries at Taiyuan had telegraphed a grave warning to British Minister Sir Claude MacDonald: "Outlook very black ... secret orders from Throne to encourage Boxers." A month earlier, the American ambassador had been warned by missionaries in Shantung that "unless Legations combine pressure, Americans consider situation almost hopeless."

MacDonald did not seem to think the implications of Tz'u-hsi's edict were worth reporting. He did send London a written report, which took two months to arrive, mentioning the proclamation, but felt that in view of the divergence of opinion as to its effects he did not at the time propose to raise the issue with the Tsungli Yamen. He did, however, join the Americans, French, Germans and Italians 10 days later in a protest against the Empress Dowager's proclamation. The protest had no effect.

Yesterday's youth gangs had now become a recognizable force. Red scarves were wound around shaven heads, red coats blazed and red bands adorned wrists and ankles. Banners, embroidered with the Boxers' anti-barbarian slogan, waved fiercely in the hot dry winds outside Peking. Warning placards were replaced with the fierce command that all Christian converts should be killed and all churches burned to the ground. One placard read: "Everyone who intends to spare someone, or to disobey our order by concealing Christian converts ... will be burned to death to prevent his impeding our programme."[8]

On the surface, Tz'u-hsi still tolerated the missionaries, saying that doctors like Leonora should live as they pleased, "making such medicines as they desire — and teach their own religion — but to people who are receptive." To this reasonable phrase she added the confusing caveat that as she was not receptive, the foreigners remained "the curse of China today."[9] Tz'u-hsi wavered to the point of absurdity, because she then issued instructions that although China should be strengthened against the foreigners — by the Boxers if necessary — Christianity and foreigners should be tolerated and accorded their legitimate treaty rights.

At the beginning of this new century, the Empress Dowager found herself surrounded by Manchu princes and dukes who had done nothing all their lives but loll in their palaces, smoke a bit of opium, and frequent flower boats, or pleasure houses. These aristocrats had ignored their education and become coarse, crude and ignorant of the world around them. This motley but bejewelled assembly, led by the decadent Prince Tuan, pressured her to enrol the Boxers as government troops.

The Tsungli Yamen, once a balanced and rational house of lords, now teetered on the brink of the idiotic. Prince Ch'ing, weak and dishonest, headed the house; Shih-to, who had never done anything of note, still drank at the royal trough, and the somewhat meek Jung-lu sat as presiding adviser. Han Chinese such as Li Hung-chang, who had traditionally provided a balance of opinion, quietly bided his time in the south as Viceroy of Kwangtun and Kwangsi. The moderate Yu-Lu, Li's successor in Tientsin, wrung his hands in vain.

In early February, Li Hung-chang summoned Leonora south to attend his daughter in Nanking. Because the doctor was still a bit shaky from her malaria, Alex went along, but returned to Tientsin almost immediately. Considering the daily reports that the aging Viceroy received from Peking, the summons may well have been a final effort to spirit his friends away from danger and into his jurisdiction. After a few weeks in Nanking, however, Leonora insisted on returning to her hospital in an ever-more-troubled Tientsin.[10]

By April Leonora, Alex and the few remaining Westerners in the city were surrounded by the Boxers, joined by Imperial troops. The populace of Tientsin blamed the misery of the drought not on the Empress Dowager, but on the evil influence of the foreigners. On the 16th, Leonora's colleague Dr. G.P. Smith of the London Missionary Society wrote that the Boxer movement was spreading like wildfire, and he was quite certain that people in authority were secretly encouraging it. It was, he wrote, "having a prejudicial effect on our work [and] the Christians are being threatened." Smith echoed the common sentiment that if only they could get three days' heavy rain "to enable the poor farmers to sow their crops, it would work wonders. The want of rain is being blamed on the Christians." But the hot white Chinese sun shone on relentlessly, day after rainless day.

From Peking, Sarah Pike Conger wrote "[the Boxers] believe that the "foreign devils" have bewitched their gods, poisoned their wells, brought sickness upon their children, and are striving to ruin them completely. ... They claim that many thousands of spirit soldiers will come down, sweep away the 'foreign devils,' and set the Chinese free." The Boxers, added Sarah, were firm in their belief that no bullets or other weapons could harm them, and the Chinese soldiers, believing them, told her "No good to shoot; can't kill them." On May 1, she wrote that "this week the Boxer work grows darker and darker. It comes nearer and nearer and is now within Peking."[11]

Handbills, depicting foreigners as pigs or goats to be devoured by the Chinese Tiger, began to appear on village as well as city walls. (Christians were often drawn as pigs because the character for one of the Chinese terms for Christianity [*T'ien chu Chiao*] was written in characters that also meant "The Squeak of the Heavenly Pig.") A Commandant Harfeld, in his *Opinion chinoise sur les Barbares d'Occident*, translated one of the handbills:

> The scandalous conduct of Christians and barbarians is irritating our Gods and Geniuses, hence the many scourges we are suffering ... (Railways) are disturbing the terrestrial dragon. ... The red liquid which keeps dripping from the iron snake (rusty water from telegraph wires) is nothing but the blood of the outraged spirits of the air. ... The missionaries extract the eyes, marrow and heart of the dead in order to make medicaments...As for the children received in orphanages, they are killed and their intestines are used to change lead into silver and to make precious remedies."[12]

The Empress Dowager was in a decidedly uncomfortable position. Reformers such as the scholar K'ang Yu-wei roared in the newspapers that she had murdered her co-empress, slept with a "spurious eunuch," and caused Emperor Hsien-feng to die of spleen and indignation. The peasants blamed Tz'u-hsi, with her direct line to heaven, for not intervening with the gods to save their crops.

The situation deteriorated. Li Hung-chang's failure to negotiate better terms in the Sino-Japanese peace treaty had exacted a harsh new taxation of the poor, in order to help pay reparation fees. The foreign steamship and telegraph lines and the railway had taken work from thousands of junk captains, coolies and couriers. The missionaries' use of Western magic (science) as a way of selling the One True God had raised rural Chinese hackles for half a century and more. And always the blithe assumption of superiority held by businessmen, diplomats and missionaries alike, fanned the flames of hatred.

In his May 10, 1900, report to London, Alex noted that although trouble was indeed on their doorstep, Leonora and he did not intend to avail themselves of the board's permission to return home on furlough, even though Alex wanted desperately to go. Leonora was now more than healthy enough to travel — if not to England, at least, like the other missionaries, to safety in Japan, North America or Australia. There were few patients these days, but as usual, when she refused to budge, Alex would not move without her.

On the same day an article appeared in the *North China Daily News*, courtesy of a "native Correspondent." This man, a minor official who was well respected in the foreign community, said:

> "I write in all seriousness and sincerity to inform you that there is a great secret scheme, having for its aim to crush all foreigners ... and wrest back the territories 'leased' to them ... all Chinese of the upper class know this, and those who count foreigners among their friends have warned ... but have to my own knowledge been rather laughed at for their pains than thanked."[13]

Depending on their location, the missionaries remained divided in their opinions. If the drought was blamed on Christians in Tientsin, quite the opposite held true in Peking, where Tz'u-hsi was held solely responsible. Four days after Alex's communiqué to London, his LMS colleague Stonehouse, based in Peking, wrote "the city is full of 'Boxers' & their threatenings are many & varied." In fact, he said, their "exercising" took place directly opposite the legations' front gates every night. Perhaps because of Claude MacDonald's refusal to recognize the danger, Stonehouse still remained strangely unaffected. "This is no cause for serious alarm to us, though they have already fixed a date when we are to be demolished," he wrote almost gaily. "The movement is now utilized by the Government to distract the attention of the people from thinking of the long drought we have had, & which drought was attributed to the wickedness of the Empress."

On May 17, three villages were destroyed and 61 converts massacred just 150 kilometres from Peking. The next day a London Mission chapel was reduced to smoking rubble.

Then the Boxers, who had been keeping Tientsin under siege, entered the old city. Historians Zhang Li and Liu Jian-tang reported that they first attacked and burnt churches because they knew quite clearly that churches were the base camps for the imperialists to commit crimes, the strongholds to aggress on China and the target that the people hated."[14]

Because of the siege, Leonora knew that foreign medicine was facing a much greater obstacle than she had yet encountered. Because of the Boxers' threats, reported her LMS colleague Dr. Smith, "very few country people come to our dispensary, the attendance is less than in 1/2 of the corresponding time last year." Able-bodied Christian converts were, however, living in mortal terror. As the conflagration heated up, Leonora and Alex were trying their best to protect native Christians, "many of whom are flocking to our compounds." The missionaries set to work erecting barricades of flour sacks, old oil drums, even church pews. Food would soon become critical.[14]

On May 19, Bishop Favier of Peking warned the diplomats that the anti-Christian propaganda was "only a cloak for the wholesale slaughter of foreigners." Bowing to the Bishop's considerable clout, Sir Claude MacDonald agreed to send to Tientsin for more guards.[15] This naturally left Tientsin less defended.

Alex's colleagues in Peking provided London with "précis notes" that characterized the continuing assumption that the Boxers were nothing more than a temporary nuisance. "1) Increasing power of the Boxers in Peking. 2) The British Minister took steps to stop the annoyance to the mission. He believes the danger has passed away for the present." Although no one dared say it at the time, Sir Claude MacDonald could not have been more wrong.

In Tientsin, the moderate Viceroy Yu-lu tried in vain to convince the Boxers that they should be a defensive rather than an aggressive force. He failed miserably. By the end of the month, the youth gangs were attacking railways, burning converts' houses and occupying the opulent quarters from which many Westerners had fled. Viceroy Yu-lu telegraphed to Peking that "persuasion can no longer disperse them. The commanders, if hesitant and tolerant, will certainly [invite] calamities."[16]

On May 28, two railroad bridges were destroyed on a branch road. The village of Fentai, including train station, cars, shops and the Empress Dowager's private rail car were all burned. Sarah Conger reported that urgent notes and frantic visitors were keeping her husband more than busy. The foreign ministers again visited the Tsungli Yamen and wrote letters, earnestly and beseechingly asking aid of the government in suppressing these outrages. In addition, they asked formal permission to bring their own guards to the Legations. The Yamen at first positively refused to grant the request, but relented at 2 am on May 31. Ambassador Conger telegraphed Admiral Kempff in Tientsin, who cabled back: "Leave on special train, three hundred and fifty strong."

At 8 pm that day, 337 smartly dressed international troops arrived at the Peking railway station. They were soon followed by 89 German and Austrian soldiers. Lulled into a sense of security, Sir Claude MacDonald cabled Admiral Seymour in Tientsin. "No more ships wanted at Taku [forts, in Tientsin] unless matters become more complicated which I do not think they will."[17] The legations were now protected by twice the number of foreign guards that the Chinese government had officially permitted.

On June 4, both the telegraph line and the railway between Tientsin and Peking were destroyed. On the 7th two British missionaries were murdered just 64 kilometres south of Peking. On the 9th, the diplomats' prized racecourse went up in a furious blaze. This final outrage was felt more keenly, more personally by the diplomats than any missionary accounts of atrocities against native Christians. It was, wrote Col. Peter Fleming in his *Siege at Peking*, "the straw that broke the camel's back." Sir Claude MacDonald cabled for more reinforcements from Tientsin.

With fewer and fewer troops to defend it, Leonora's city was desperately trying to survive the repeated onslaughts of the Boxers. The stench of scorched earth and rotting bodies filled the city's parched air. Flies droned ceaselessly around the carcasses, laying their eggs in each gaping wound. Already some corpses were white with seething waves of maggots. From beyond the compound walls, high-pitched screams of 'Burn Burn Burn! Kill Kill Kill!' raised the hair on the back of everyone's necks. One Tientsin missionary had written with fatality, "we are practically in a state of war. The long-foreseen crisis is upon us. ... Any moment may reveal that the Empress has decided to order [the troops] openly to join the mob ... we are calmed by the certainty that prayer is being offered for us and for poor China."

Because Tientsin was besieged, missionaries from the interior were pouring into the legations in Peking. "All foreigners are leaving their compounds and missions and going to the Legations and to the Methodist mission," wrote Sarah Conger. The mission where the young Leonora had first lived, back in 1877, was described by Mrs. Conger as the largest, nearest, and best fortified of all. As for the legations, the ambassador's wife had "our best storeroom filled with extras — much flour, corn meal, beans, rice, and sugar; besides chickens and other supplies. ...We filled our coal bin and bought large kangs holding great quantities of water."

The foreign compounds in Tientsin were deplorably ill protected by what was left of the international troops. All day and all night, the acrid smell of smoke from the few cannons permeated the compounds. Leonora and Alex's home was attacked, as were the homes of their absent colleagues. The Boxers razed a missionary-built temperance hall, called "Little White House," just across the street from the Astor Hotel. The one relatively safe place to hide was in the wine cellar of the hotel itself.

On June 9, the Emperor, the Empress Dowager and their court moved back from the Summer Palace to the Forbidden City. On the 10th, Admiral Seymour left Tientsin with a trainload of 2,129 soldiers and sailors.[18] They were expected to reach Peking that night. One hundred and thirty kilometres away, the Peking diplomats, unaware of the wrecked railway lines, stood in vain at the silent station. They did not know that Seymour, who had passed friendly General Nieh's Imperial army on the way, had been driven back to Tientsin by a monstrous force of Boxers and village hangers-on. "Please believe me," Seymour wrote to Peking, "we are doing our utmost to get on. ... should these [railway] obstacles prove insuperable, I will consider if we can march to your relief."[19]

That afternoon, Sugiyama, the Japanese chancellor, returned to the Peking train-station to see if Seymour had arrived. The story as reported by *Times* correspondent George Morrison and his colleagues said that the chancellor was dragged brutally from his cart and hacked to pieces in front of an appreciative crowd. Most of his corpse was left in the gutter, but his heart was cut out and sent to General Tung Fu-hsiang, whose troops were the Japanese diplomat's assassins. In reality, Sugiyama was stoned to death.[20]

On June 12, the Boxers entered Peking in force. The foreign guard cleared the legation area and stationed guns and men to guard the inhabitants. On the 18th, The Boxers had burned all the mission buildings, including the Catholic mission, Nantang, which had been built in 1600. Pethick, Li Hung-chang's longtime secretary, led 20 Russians and 10 American marines in order to rescue the missionaries and converts at Nantang. "Four of our men brought over four hundred refugees past this Legation," wrote Sarah Conger, "... many hungry, burned, wounded, and slashed. ... Such fortitude I never beheld, as these people manifested during the dressing of their wounds. No shrinking, nor cry of suffering ... our sincere sympathy was with them."

But tragedy struck even the pro-Boxer element. In the Forbidden City, the Empress Dowager and her ladies watched in despair as the glorious Ch'ien Men gateway to the Tartar City burned fiercely into the night. The harsh winds of Peking then swept the sparks inward, igniting Peking's richest quarter. Shops containing priceless artifacts, furs, jewels and rare silks produced spectacular explosions in the tinder-dry air. The Boxers were out of control, and Tz'u-hsi knew it.

Endnotes

1. Council for World Missionary Archives, Day Missions Library, Yale University. London Missionary Society Records. Box H-2139. 1900.
2. Frazer Smith, James, Reverend, MD, CM. *Life's Waking Part*. Toronto: Thomas Nelson and Sons, Limited, 1937, p. 257.
3. Warner, Marina. *The Dragon Empress: Life and Times of Tz'u-hsi, 1835-1908, Empress Dowager of China*. London: Cardinal, 1974, p. 209.
4. Fairbank, John K. *The Missionary Enterprise in China and America*. Cambridge, Mass.: Harvard University Press, 1974, p. 366.
5. Ibid., p. 366.
6. Conger, Sarah Pike. *Letters from China*. Chicago: A.C. McClurg & Co., 1910, pp. 40-42.
7. Fleming, Peter. *The Siege at Peking*. New York: Dorset Press, New York, 1990, pp. 54-55.
8. Warner, *The Dragon Empress*, p. 217.
9. Ibid., p. 217.
10. Council for World Missionary Archives, Day Missions Library, Yale University. London Missionary Society Records. Box H-2139. 1900.

11. Conger, *Letters from China*, pp. 90-91.
12. Warner, *The Dragon Empress*, p. 218.
13. Fleming, *The Siege at Peking*, p. 63.
14. Council for World Missionary Archives, Day Missions Library, Yale University. London Missionary Society Records. Box H-2139. 1900.
15. Warner, *The Dragon Empress*, p. 224.
16. Ibid., p. 224.
17. Fleming, *The Siege at Peking*, pp. 54-55.
18. Ibid., p. 75.
19. Ibid., p. 100.
20. Conger, *Letters from China*, p. 100.

Chapter nineteen

Tientsin burns
1900

For nation shall rise against nation, and kingdom against kingdom.
— Matthew 24:7

Admiral Seymour's force comprised British, German, Russian, French, American, Japanese, Italian and Austrian soldiers, sailors and marines. They had seven field guns and 10 machine guns. Aware that the railway line had been broken at Lofa, about halfway to Peking, they had taken with them a gang of coolies with materials for repairing the line. Just after noon, they had run into General Nieh Shih-cheng, whose army, trained by Li Hung-chang's aide-de-camp General Hannekon, had recently fought against the Boxers. Although Nieh Shih-cheng had been sharply reprimanded for fighting the Boxers, he continued his stance by allowing Seymour to continue his rescue mission.

The line at Lofa was easily repaired, but a little further on, the Langfang station and its water tanks were found destroyed. The engines were watered well enough with buckets, but the troops began to suffer from dehydration owing to the intense heat. Some collapsed in their tracks, adding to the rumour that all wells had been poisoned. On the third day of Seymour's mission, about 200 Boxers attacked with no sign of fear of hesitation. Although this first attack was thwarted within 20 minutes, it was followed by others of greater ferocity. General Nieh disappeared, and Seymour's troops were perilously divided, guarding the many stations en route to Peking. Carrying the wounded added to his considerable difficulties, and further progress by rail was now considered impossible. His only alternative was to head back to Yangstun and head upriver on a fleet of four requisitioned junks. It was now June 17. One week had passed since Seymour's troops had set out for a "few hours' journey" to Peking. At Yangtsun, the troops again heard the muted boom of artillery fire coming from Tientsin. On the 18th, the German contingent at Langfang was attacked by a major force of 4,000 regular Chinese troops. The Government had joined the Boxers.[1]

This disastrous development had been felt by Leonora and Alex two days earlier, when the Boxers had invaded Tientsin's foreign settlements. Their total garrison, including 1,600 Russians who had arrived too late to join Seymour's troops, consisted of 2,400 men with the unenviable task of defending an 8-kilometre perimeter. Admiral Seymour now returned to Tientsin with cartloads of wounded. Leonora's hospital and all others were commandeered by the armed forces. Leonora found herself tending the wounded night and day, alternating between treating her own flocks and working side by side with military doctors, all of whom were men. Although nothing is reported of their relationships, it is likely that some military doctors would first have balked at a woman assisting them, but as things went from bad to worse, her surgical skill and knowledge of Chinese would become most welcome.

The allied forces retrenched and, with the help of the recently arrived Russians, seized the Taku forts. Viceroy Jung-Lu, probably fearing for his head, reported this fact to Peking. Mrs. Conger, the American ambassador's wife, reported that the Tsungli Yamen presented all the legations with (in substance) the following message:

> "We learn that foreign troops are to fire upon our forts near Tientsin, hence we break off all diplomatic relations with your Government and ask that you leave Peking in twenty-four hours. No further protection will be given by us."

The foreign ministers sent a reply that it was out of the question to go, and requested an audience with the Tsungli Yamen. With no reply forthcoming, the German minister, Baron von Ketteler, decided go alone, because he had other business to discuss with the Yamen. "He started with his interpreter, two mounted mafoos, and two chairs," wrote Sarah Conger. "They had not gone ... three-quarters of a mile before they were attacked. One mafoo rushed back to the German Legation; the other went to the Tsung Li [sic] Yamen. The interpreter was badly wounded and taken to the Methodist mission ... Baron Von Ketteler, was shot through the head ... they found only the two chairs, badly crushed."[2]

The Empress Dowager, now more frightened than furious, made plans to evacuate the Imperial palace. In Tientsin, because he had yet to hear otherwise, an overly optimistic Alex reported to London that things were fine elsewhere: "Your telegram enquiring as to the safety of our missionaries came a day or two ago. ... We are in constant communication with all our stations. Doubtless you will hear by this mail from Peking. I hear that all foreigners are in the British

Legation. ... The relief guard should be in Peking soon [but] there is no telegraph communication with the capital at present."

In Peking, the foreigners had indeed been driven into the final refuge of the British legation. The Methodist compound, where the young Leonora had arrived from Canada so many years ago, was now considered too isolated to be safe, and was ordered evacuated. Some 5,000 people now crowded into the legation compound, including diplomats, merchants, missionaries, servants and Chinese Christian converts. Sarah Conger reported that "Austrian, Dutch and Belgian Legations have been burned, also the Imperial Customs, and all the missions, including the Methodist mission." The Dutch Legation, just west of the American one, had presented a new peril when "the wind took the flames up to our very walls, even burning the quarters of the American marines." Luckily the wind changed and the American legation was saved.

The final cable out of Peking came from "a committee of American missionaries," which was blown up on the front page of the *New York World*. It said: "Arouse the Christian World Immediately to Our Peril. Should This Arrive too Late, Avenge Us!"[3]

A group of Canadians at Honan, led by fire-and-brimstone Reverend Jonathan Goforth, had received a message from Tientsin's British Consul commanding all to flee for their lives, but, Alex noted, "our Consul Mr. Carlos, who has given the very greatest help to us ... cannot urge our missionaries in the interior to leave their stations so we have wired to both our southern stations 'Tientsin un-approachable': if in doubt go south."

Just days before the British consul's message arrived at Honan, a small group of Canadian missionaries had departed on a houseboat for their summer vacation. About half way to Tientsin, they received Alex's warning to approach no further. Abandoning their houseboats, the missionaries escaped through a section of Shangtung where the rebels were still held in check by officials. After enduring many hardships, all arrived safely in Chefoo.

On June 24, Alex's colleague, Reverend Lees, wrote that a relief force had entered Tientsin the night before after a week of bombardment. The loss of life, among Europeans at least, had been minimal, but all the mission chapels, except those in the settlement, had been reduced to smoking rubble. Leonora, like people in the legations in Peking, began to rely on supplies from other concessions and from the foreign hotels. Bolts of new cotton, sheeting, pillow casing, new tablecloths, napkins and towels were turned into the common store. Bed-nets, pillows, mattresses, blankets — even dresses and skirts — were turned into bandages. Water was becoming precious.

By mid-summer all communication with Tientsin had effectively been cut off, and the Canadians at Honan were left to cope as best they could. Jonathan Goforth's missionaries were in fact all set to flee, but at the last minute they were frustrated by the Chinese district chief who refused to cooperate in an evacuation. Goforth told him "we knew the Treaties and that he must grant us an escort. ... The foreign powers have seized Taku and a settlement of this trouble must come."[4] His manner seemed to work. On June 28, the Canadians were on their way — not to Tientsin, but south to Shanghai.

The Honan missionaries began their long march huddled in clumsy freight carts covered with straw mats, the mats being their only protection from the merciless Chinese sun. Rumbling and creaking through the dust, they proceeded to the river, where they joined forces with three British engineers and their escort. At this point, the group decided to split into two contingents, in the hope that at least one might get through in safety. On July 8, Goforth's party was suddenly attacked by two bands of "several hundreds" armed with swords, spears and guns, "one lot standing in a body waiting for us, and the other lot ... ready to attack us in the rear." As the Canadians, who all survived, consisted of a tiny group of five men, six women and five children, with three revolvers among them, Goforth's "several hundreds" may have been somewhat of an exaggeration.

Attacking in a rush, he reported, one band began pelting stones at the mule carts, but the straw mats kept the missiles from penetrating. Goforth claimed that the Chinese killed some of the mules and maimed others before turning on the missionaries. (This seems unlikely, because the mules were worth their weight in gold to any Chinese. The mules were probably stolen.) By his own account, Goforth received nine wounds on his arms and hands and eight blows with clubs, but his most severe wound came from a sword blow to the back of the neck (he miraculously escaped decapitation when the sword bounced off his pith helmet). Canadian Dr. Percy Leslie's right hand was almost severed at the wrist, while Dr. Mackenzie and the Reverend John Griffith received ugly sword slashes. Griffith had one of the revolvers, but it had been broken by a stone in the initial attack. Goforth reported that Griffith found a large club and fought "like a hero" with his back to the cart. As luck would have it, the attackers began to quarrel among themselves as they started to loot the missionaries' belongings. The Canadians seized this opportunity to escape, leaving all their worldly goods behind.

Percy Leslie was so badly wounded that the missionaries feared he would bleed to death. In addition to 15 sword wounds, his wrist and kneecap were broken. Dr. Jean Dow staunched the bleeding with bandages she had made from the missionaries' clothing. Stripped of wedding rings, watches and most of their outer clothing during the attack, the party, dragging Leslie in the lone salvaged cart, managed to get a safe distance before they succumbed to the incredible heat. After a little while, when they came out of their daze, they realized the Goforths were missing. Retracing their steps, the Canadians were guided to the house of a friendly Muslim, where they found a badly wounded Jonathan Goforth resting on a straw mat.

Their host, though sympathetic, told them to hurry onward, as he was justifiably afraid of the consequences of harbouring foreigners. On the road again, they were almost immediately surrounded by a "boisterous, jeering mob." As they proceeded south, they were held up again and again by robbers who tore open the women's clothing to find concealed jewellery and silver. Finally they were rescued by cavalry that had been sent by the official at Nan-Yang-fu, about eight miles south. At the city, the exhausted missionaries were forced into a stifling little room where they were put on display, remaining for hours with neither food nor water. When Goforth protested to the Yamen, he was informed that the group would have to move on at the curious hour of midnight.

The missionaries had justifiable suspicions about a midnight escort by some unknown soldiers. As they left the city, Reverend Griffith, who had left the carts to "reconnoitre" with nine-year-old Paul Goforth, found himself shoeless and abandoned in the dark. After trudging along a river bed for some hours, the man and the boy found the sandy soil so inviting that they curled up for a few hours' sleep. When their absence was detected, the others stopped for consultation and held a midnight prayer-meeting for their missing brethren, then shouted into the darkness in the hope of hearing responding "halloos!" Although his son was missing, Goforth as leader decided that it would be impossibly dangerous to turn back. At this point, the soldiers "stealthily slipped off the carts, and disappeared into the darkness."

A little while later, the carters themselves stopped, refusing to go any farther. Then the almost incredible happened in the form of an unknown friend who appeared out of nowhere to order the carters, in tones of great authority, to stick to the bargain and take the missionaries out of Honan. The strange friend stayed with the cortege for some distance. He was later described as a miraculous "Gift from God" by the tattered refugees.

The party, now bloody and ragged, were reduced to begging for food and water. One Chinese man, who had come to rob, seemed struck by their plight and instead led them through three different spots of danger, protecting the Goforth's amah, or nanny, who, as a Chinese Christian, was in even more peril than the foreigners.

Hot and tired, the missing Griffith and Paul Goforth were now stripped down to only their trousers. They were also exceedingly hungry. Both Griffith and Paul were scarcely able to walk. Griffith later wrote "my own feet were so blistered and stone bruised and pierced with thorns that it was painful to even touch them on the ground." Happily, that night a faithful servant appeared and reunited the two refugees with their joyous families.

An official account of the separation of Griffith and Paul later claimed that this occurrence actually saved the lives of the Canadians. As Griffith suspected, the soldiers were indeed out to kill the party, but "it was all or nothing — dead men tell no tales." The churchman added that it was only his ability to convince various murderous crowds that he and Paul were not Roman Catholic that saved their lives — in fact, one man hell-bent on "braining them" with a large club disappeared, only to return with 100 Cash, which he gave to young Paul to help them on their way.

The British engineers, led by a Mr. Jamieson, now surfaced again, providing the missionaries with a welcome $400. Jamieson wired the pro-Western viceroy of Wuchang, who dispatched two gunboats and two boatloads of soldiers to Fancheng to escort the Canadians to Hankow. The engineers themselves provided a tug to help the party upstream. Said Goforth, "Our hearts were too full to speak our gratitude at the kindness we received."[5]

The other party of Canadian missionaries — the one that had split up with Goforth at the beginning of the trek — finally passed the Honan border into Hupeh Province, where they were protected by Viceroy Chang Chih-tung Houseboats conveyed them to Hankow, where they arrived July 21, exactly 24 days after they had left their homes. From Hankow, the missionaries steamed safely to Shanghai, where they offered up thanks to God in the form of a rather bureaucratic resolution.

> "Resolved that we, the members of Honan Presbytery, as our first act after the terrible events in Honan, do hereby, deliverance vouchsafed, whereby every member of the Mission, male and female, escaped safely ... do hereby solemnly reconsecrate ourselves to God's service, in behalf of the Salvation of China."[6]

Notwithstanding the resolution, most of the missionaries intelligently left for Kobe, Japan, and then home.

In Shansi and Hopeh, 136 Protestant adults, 53 children, and 54 Catholic priests and nuns were hunted down, burned alive, shot, disembowelled, and beheaded. Their heads, as per Chinese custom, were left hanging from the city walls. Of the 89 adult members of the China Inland Mission, 46 were murdered. One group[7] was beheaded right in the governor's yamen. A poignant message from the dead survived from the pen of one woman, who wrote: "I was very restless and excited while there seemed a chance of life ... but God has taken away that feeling, and now I just pray for grace to meet the terrible end bravely." Only three Canadians were in Shansi province at the time. Missionary Alec Saunders of the China Inland Mission, a friend of Goforth's, spent 49 days "wandering in deserts and mountains and vales and holes of the earth," while William Peat of the Hamilton Young Men's Christian Association and Margaret Smith of New Hamburg, Ontario, both died violently.

The Chinese Christians left behind in Honan province, if they were allowed to live, were terrorized, robbed, tortured, beaten and left destitute. There is no record of the Chinese death toll.

From a smoldering Tientsin, Alex wrote: "Dear Mr. Cousins: The military authorities have asked all ladies and children to leave Tientsin. Mrs. King is very unwilling to go away, but we may be obliged." On July 6th and again on the 11th, Alex wrote again. "Tientsin (European) has been heavily bombarded today and Mr. Lee's house only escaped being broken down by the promptness of his house coolie. ... All our houses have been hit. Mrs. Bryson, Mrs. King and I intend to remain. "

On July 11, "Just a word from this much-shelled city. Matters do not improve ... on the 8th and 9th bombardment was furious ... we know absolutely nothing of the state of matters in Peking." A sad, small, scribbled note appeared in the borders of Alex's letter: "P.S. an American lady doctor and 2 American missionaries still remain on besides us. All others have gone away."

On a lighter note, when the telegraph line between Tientsin and Peking had been cut on June 14, Li Hung-chang's former aide-de-camp, General Hannekon, made plans to erect a provisional long-distance line to help the foreigners remain in touch. Leading a squad of the (Austrian) Victorian Navy, he had completed the dangerous work of erecting the poles by mid-July, but found he had no insulators for the line. Proper insulation material was nowhere to be found, he wrote. "In disappointment, we decided to use the necks of beer bottles instead. ... We got several carts of bottles within several days [from the Astor and Queen's hotels] ... rapidly, we set up the line and put it to use." This "Bottle-Neck Line," which was used to send cipher telegrams at first, became a lifeline for the besieged British legation in Peking.[8]

By August, every mission station in China had been evacuated and 3,000 people had converged in Shanghai and Hankow.

Still in Tientsin, on August 6, Alex wrote: "We heard yesterday that the Chinese re-commenced firing on the British Legation on the 2nd, also that the Empress Dowager had ... sent provisions to the Legation, but last week the Vice President of one of the Boards was killed by the Boxers because he tried to send provisions to the foreigners ... if that is true we fear the worst as regards our friends in Peking. The relief force has only got 1/4 of the distance to Peking from here. They have twice severely defeated the Chinese troops — who greatly outnumber the allied forces."

On the 13th, the Russian troops ignored agreements with the other allied troops and stormed the gates at Peking, suffering heavy losses but finally gaining admittance to the capital. On the 14th, the British and Americans joined them. On the 15th, the Japanese troops, after hard fighting, entered the city after dark. The besieged in the legations first heard a series of dull booms, then a sound like tapping quickly with one finger on the table. "The scene in the British Legation was indescribable," wrote Sir Claude MacDonald. "Those who, tired out, had fallen asleep were wakened by these unwonted sounds, and there was much cheering and shaking of hands. The enemy, too, had heard it. For a moment there was silence; then the rifle-fire broke out more angry and deafening that before, instantly responded to by the rattle of our sharp-shooters and the grunt of the five-barrelled Nordenfelt."[9] The siege of Peking had lasted 55 days. Sixty-six foreigners were killed and more than 150 people wounded; two adults and six babies had died. Chinese casualties were not reported.

By August 30, Tientsin was safe. Alex and Leonora asked London for financial help for the many Christian refugees who, unlike the foreigners, had no hope of compensation for their terrible losses of life and property. "Mrs. King still stays on here," he reported. In spite of the constant bombardment and building of sandbags, "she has been able to do a little medical work all the time of the siege." Perhaps because she obviously loved a challenge, Leonora had enjoyed better health that summer than she had for five years. "Of course," wrote her husband, "the military occupation of Tientsin & Peking will continue all winter, but we ... will rejoice when we cease to be under martial law."

On September 24, Alex's colleague, LMS missionary Mrs. Bryson, took over the letter writing to London, reporting that Alex now had been ill for three weeks with a severe attack of typhoid malarial fever. The devoted Leonora attended him throughout, although several friends helped with night nursing. Still Leonora did not, apparently, feel that Alex's illness was enough reason to relocate to friendlier climes. "Mrs. King has no intention of leaving Tientsin even after his recovery," wrote the unhappy missionary.

On October 20, Alex wrote: "I am just recovering from the only serious illness in my life." He had started to rally when a relapsing fever "nearly finished me up. I know for a fact," he said lovingly, "if I had not had both an excellent nurse and a physician of no ordinary skill in the house (my wife) I could never have pulled through the past few weeks." Alex noted carefully that he would be most willing to leave, after all the carnage of war and his own frightening illness, but Leonora was again digging in her heels. "I was very anxious to taking my furlough last spring, as granted by the Board," he said, "but Mrs. King refused to leave China. ... She is in better health than she has been for many years. She says it took her 2 years to recover from her journey to England 10 years ago. She is also the worst sailor that ever set foot on a steamboat — her Canadian home is broken up & she couldn't stand the Canadian winter as she did — she positively refuses to go to England to live."

Alex continued with some optimism, tempered with a resignation born of long association with Leonora and her Chinese protector: "... I think I shall get her to leave Tientsin (for the South of Europe or America) for a time next spring: although Li Hung Chang [sic] who was passing through Tientsin lately hoped she would go on with her medical work among Chinese women — saying if her usual Government supplies were not soon resumed he would see that she did not suffer from want of $ to carry on her work (and to that work she is wedded)."

It had been the siege of the British Legation in Peking that finally aroused the world to the fact that the Dowager Empress supported this full-scale revolt. Sadly for the foreigners in the north but luckily for those further south, the Manchu government was in such decline that many viceroys ignored Tz'u-hsi's xenophobic edicts. The Boxers had remained confined to the northern Honan, Shansi, Shantung and Leonora's province of Chihli.

Tientsin was now, to our history's eternal shame, being looted indiscriminately by allied troops. One young man from Brantford, Ontario, who had joined the American marines, wrote: "You can't imagine what this city looks like. ... Dead (Chinese) are lying around the streets, and every day the river receives a consignment of their bodies. ... Pigtails are scattered all around. ... I would send a silk robe if I could put it in a letter, but as I can't you can keep this bit of ribbon as a souvenir of the fall of Tien Tsin [sic]."

Endnotes

1. Fleming, Peter. *The Siege at Peking*. New York: Dorset Press, 1990, pp. 75-78.
2. Conger, Sarah Pike. *Letters from China*. Chicago: A.C. McClurg & Co., 1910, p. 109.
3. Fairbank, John K., ed. *The Missionary Enterprise in China and America*. Cambridge, Mass.: Harvard University Press, 1974, p. 273.
4. Forsythe, R.C., quoting Goforth, J. The China Martyrs of 1900. From: Stursberg, Peter. *The Golden Hope*. Toronto: United Church Publishing House, 1987, p. 49.
5. Stursberg, *The Golden Hope*, p. 53.
6. Frazer Smith, James, Reverend, MD, CM, *Life's Waking Part*. Toronto: Thomas Nelson and Sons, Limited, 1937, p. 263.
7. Austin, Alvyn J. *Saving China - Canadian Missionaries in the Middle Kingdom*, 1888-1959. Toronto: University of Toronto Press, 1986, p. 76.
8. Liu Jiantang and Tian Yutang, eds. *Astor Hotel Sightseeing Over a Century*. Tianjin, People's Republic of China: Tianjin People's Publishing House, 1993, pp. 266, 457. Quotes from "Tientsin Customs: Report from 1892 to 1902," Note that shortly thereafter, this became the first telephone line from Tientsin to Peking, and was used for three years. It was the beginning of modern telephone systems in China.
9. Fleming, *The Siege at Peking*, p. 205.

Map of Peking

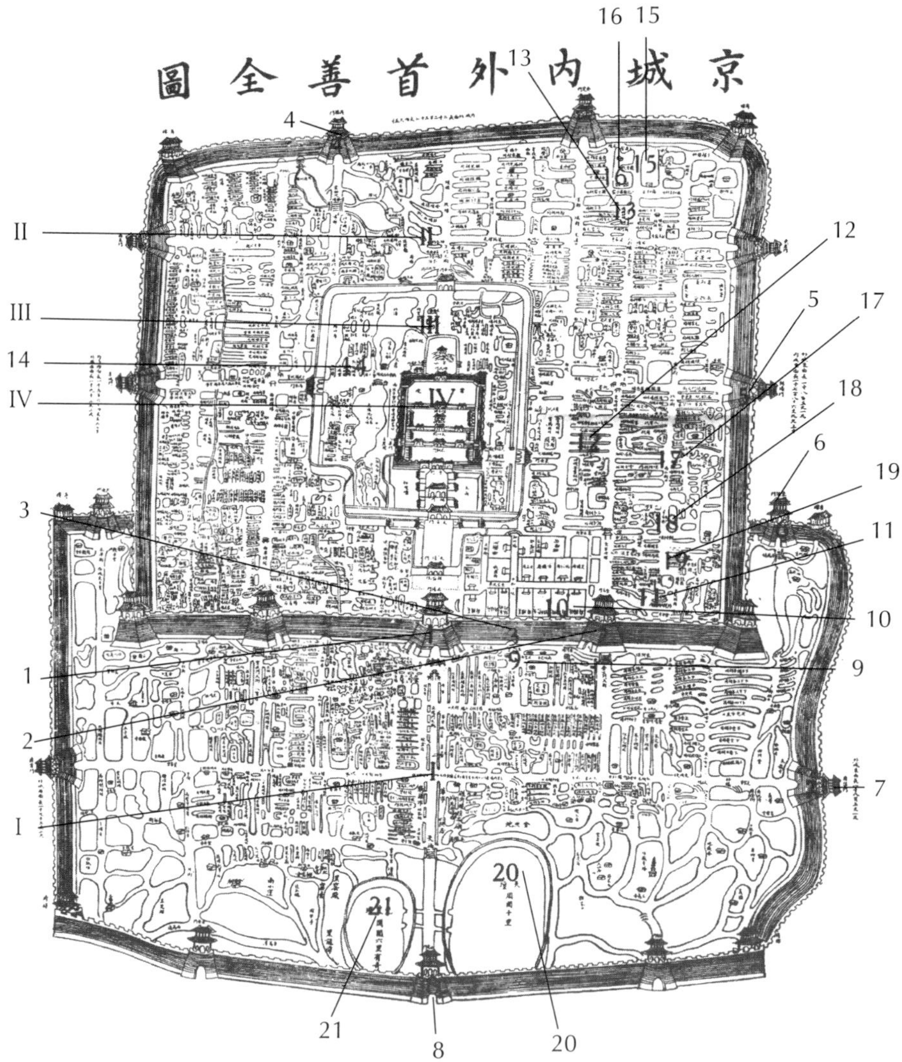

I- Native City
II- Tartar City
III- Imperial City
IV- Forbidden City
1- Ch'ienmen
2- Hatamen
3- Wall between the two gates fortified by the besieged
4- Te-shengmen (court fled through this gate August 15, 1900)
5- Ch'i Huamen (Russian and Japanese relief entered at this gate in 1900)
6- Tungpienmen (the gate through which the Americans entered in 1900)
7- Shakuomen (where the British entered in 1900)
8- Yungtingmen (gate leading into the city from the station)
9- Water Gate (here the relief troops entered the legation)
10- Legation quarters
11- Methodist Mission
12- American Board Mission
13- Presbyterian Mission
14- Peitang
15- Lama temple
16- Confucian temple
17- Tsung Li Yamen
18- Examination Halls
19- Imperial Observatory
20- Temple of Heaven, British headquarters in 1900
21- Temple of Agriculture, American headquarters in 1900

Chapter twenty

The lashback
1901

The expense of spirit in a waste of shame
Is lust in action ...
— William Shakespeare

After Tientsin and Peking had been liberated, troops, diplomats and even missionaries set about the serious business of looting. Count Witte, the Russian Ambassador, wrote: "One [Russian] lieutenant general, who had received the Cross of St George for the capture of Peking, returned to his post ... with ten trunks full of valuables from the looted ... palaces." Reverend Arthur H. Smith, who ever before and after this deplorable feeding frenzy, claimed to love and the respect the Chinese, added the suspiciously anti-Christian thought that the looting was an act of more than justifiable reprisal.

Reverend Smith wrote detachedly that the British were "most scientific" in their looting — the ancestral tablets of the Ch'ing dynasty being taken to the British Museum." A British officer reported: "Lady MacDonald was out with a small force left behind in Peking ... and devoted herself most earnestly to looting."[1] Sarah Conger, who repeatedly wrote that the Americans had given strict orders against looting, was devastated to find that the Imperial College was in ruins, its ancient treasures and artifacts destroyed or stolen. The Peking Observatory's valuable bronze instruments, used for more than four hundred years, were carried away, by parties unnamed.

Leonora, who was left with the medical and spiritual horrors of the siege, must have been appalled at the conduct of both allied forces and people such as William Ament and E.G. Tewksbury, who had led armed raiding parties against supposedly "Boxer" villages in retaliation. American missionary Luella Miner wrote that for all the Boxer atrocities, there had been no incidents of rape — a far cry from the allied forces' outrageous behaviour. In Peking, Sarah

Conger found lonely little coffins in abandoned Chinese palaces. The ladies of the house had committed suicide rather than be debauched by the foreigners.

"Poor China!" she wrote. "Why cannot foreigners let her alone with her own? ... my sympathy is with China. A very unpopular thing to say but it is an honest conviction" Her husband's opinions were diametrically opposed: the previous year, he had proposed that the United States take over Chihli province, including Peking, as a base in China.

After the siege, Leonora's medical work was spotty at best. Many families left for the south, and others fled to the country. Those remaining in and around Tientsin who desired to come to the dispensary were afraid to do so because the city was occupied by foreign soldiers. Her work consisted chiefly in caring for Christian converts from the LMS and other missions, and treating allied armed forces for dysentery. The Roman Catholics had closed their dispensary, and the British forces having occupied both Leonora's first (Isabella Fisher) and latest (Government Hospital for Women and Children), a number of their members probably came to her home for treatment. WFMS dispensary work was carried on in a three-room Chinese house at the back of the General Board Compound.

Dispensary buildings at Tientsin's West City had been completely destroyed, along with all their contents, including furniture, drugs and surgical instruments. The General Board temporarily used Chinese houses near the old site. The WFMS reported that no effort was made to start medical work until after the new year, when a weekly clinic began.

"The attendance was at first small but has gradually increased, a number of the patients coming from heathen homes, which leads one to hope that when order and good government are restored, we may be able to reach, and minister, to those who need healing for both body and soul," reported Dr. Iva Stevenson. "A full record of the treatments has not been kept this year, but estimating from a record of several months, the following represents the number approximately.

Dispensary patients	2,400
Patients treated in home	82
Fees	Gold $50.50

Farther afield, the missionaries at the Methodist girls' boarding school in Tsun Hua District reported that "as the days go by we are able to give more definite reports concerning the sufferings and martyrdom of our girls. ... They had gone to their homes ... when into our midst crashed the thunderbolts of the enemy. Our two faithful assistants, Hsu Hui Fang and Liu Wen Lan, suffered even unto death. For many weeks the former was hunted from place to place, was given first to one man and then to the second, was shot, and at the last was tortured. The second suffered but a few days, but suffered much. She went triumphantly Home, preaching the Gospel until they severed her head from her body. Another was killed at a place about ten miles from Tsun Hua, where all the Christians of her village had gathered. Many were carried off, others were married into heathen homes to keep them from such a fate. Some, in all probability, escaped all persecution, but how many we know not."[2]

The aftermath of the siege was much more serious when it came to eating. Much of the hoarded food had gone up in flames or been confiscated by the Boxers. Rice and flour stores were very low. In Peking, missionaries and diplomats alike were eating pony meat, after the mules had been consumed. Ambassador Conger's pony was first to go, as "the pony hated foreigners as bitterly as do the Chinese." Fuel was another major concern. Formerly, thousands of camel drivers had brought loads of coal into the cities daily. Now they came infrequently, if at all, and winter was approaching.

To make matters worse, the arrogance of the allies had only increased as a result of the Boxer troubles. If some of the actions were not so conceited, they would be laughable. One missionary woman wrote that she was most offended by a medal that had been created for survivors of the seige. On one side were depicted Europe, America and Japan trampling on the Chinese dragon. "I object to this first because it isn't true, as the dragon came out on the top side," she wrote angrily, and second, she added, "because it isn't polite."[3]

The allied forces — British, French, American, German, Russian, Japanese and Italian — were alleged to have murdered thousands more helpless people than the Boxers killed.[4] Foreign soldiers moved about a prostrate countryside, committing "robbery, assassinations, and nameless outrages ... numbers of innocent and peaceful non-combatants were slaughtered ... whole districts were ruthlessly and needless laid waste."

The Western press could pretend to excuse the troops' behaviour under the "boys will be boys" cloak, but when reports of missionaries leading looting expeditions began to emerge, it was really just too much for the reading public. Some American missionaries readily granted interviews to correspondents and sent open letters to editors, lay and religious, and to the Associated Press, as well as copies of petitions to Washington. Some of these public statements were so vindictive against the Chinese that they proved a source of embarrassment to their spokesmen and supporters in America.[5]

The missionaries had an incredibly bad sense of timing, as it was already known that mass murder and rape, as well as looting, was the order of the day. The *New York Sun* quoted an American missionary as saying "the Germans have the right idea, punish the Chinese first and treat with them later." The correspondent explained: "Such a remark from a missionary might seem a bit surprising to persons away from Peking, but expresses the common sentiment here."[6]

The editor of the *San Francisco Call* reported that this was a "sorry spectacle of the kind of Christianity that we seem to be exporting to Asia in carload lots. ... For every woman missionary sacrificed by the Boxers, 500 Chinese women have gone to torture and death. For every man ordained for martyrdom 1,000 Chinese men have atoned with their lives. For every missionary child cut down ... 100 Chinese babies have been tossed and impaled on Cossack spears. For every missionary ... compound burned or sacked value a hundredfold has been looted in Tientsin and Peking."

China's holy place, the magnificent Temple of Heaven, was now headquarters for the British army. The Americans used the Temple of Agriculture. The diplomats took tours through this and other areas previously barred to foreigners. "We saw many elegant furnishings ... jades, porcelains, brass, ivory, lacquer, bronze, wood carving, immense mirrors, brilliant decorations, embroidered hangings, fine large rugs," wrote Sarah Conger. "New scenes opened our eyes. ... Large, gorgeously decorated throne buildings ... and many other buildings with their beautiful, valuable treasures, were opened to us. ... the Japanese and Americans are protecting these treasures from vandalism." Not so, however, many private homes and palaces, which were happily looted by all and sundry.

Humorists Mark Twain and Finley Peter Dunne descended with a vengeance on the missionaries' already battered reputations. Dunne's character, "Mr. Dooley," described "the fine cillybration planned by th' mission'ries," viz. "First day, 10 A.M., prayers be the allied mission'ries; 1 P.M., massacre iv the impress an' rile fam'ly; sicond day, 10 A.M., scatthren iv the remains iv formers kings; 11 A.M., disecretarion iv graves gin'rally." Dunne also pictured missionaries "fillin' packin' cases with th' undherwear iv th' Chinese imp'ror an' th' spoons iv th' impress. Th' air was filled with cries iv "Hinnery, won't yet set on this trunk? I can't get th' lid down since ye put in that hateful idol."

Twain himself attacked W.S. Ament of the American Board of Missions, who had used his particular knowledge of Peking to loot the wealthiest mansions. Sir Robert Hart, Inspector-General of (Chinese) Maritime Customs, defended the missionary, saying he had been set apart by the legation authorities to take charge of whatever looted property was brought in for the use of the legations — "a tribute to his honesty and capacity."

The pinnacle of arrogant self-righteousness was reached in an article entitled *The Ethics of Looting*, written by the celebrated missionary-author Gilbert

Reid and published in *Forum* magazine. Reid actually apologized for not having personally looted more. Loot was to him simply the spoils of war, and if the Chinese did not want to be looted, they should not have started the war![7]

Compared with the armed forces, merchants and diplomats, only a minuscule number of missionaries engaged in looting. But rather than rest quietly on that plausible defence, mission spokesmen were compelled to seek complete public vindication, and in so doing, only further stained their already tarnished image. They would have been far better off following the example of Inspector General Sir Robert Hart, who, in his first public statement after arriving home, suggested that "those who say the least now will be in a better position to talk later on." The Methodist West China Mission, which was never in great danger, discouraged its people from speaking out, at least until the next year when things had calmed down. It then published, in great detail, the death of its first martyr, an itinerant Bible seller. The Canadian Presbyterian Church was especially reluctant to let the Jonathan Goforth's Honan group speak out, and sent 10 eyewitnesses to isolated stations in British Columbia to keep them out of the clutches of reporters until things died down.

Goforth, however, could not keep quiet. In Toronto, he "thrilled" an audience with his thundering oratory and tales of adventure, but a *Toronto Daily Star* reporter caught his real meaning by printing the following:

> "All we require is that the powers shall give the governors and mandarins to understand that our work is sacred, and our persons sacred, and we ask no special favours whatsoever.' If missions are to be established by gun-boats and field-guns and the sacredness of the missionaries' person and worked forced upon the recognition of rulers who are adverse to them, the heathen mind might regard these things as 'special favours.'"

In the ruins of Tientsin, the Isabella Fisher and Leonora's Government Hospital for Women and Children emerged fairly unscathed, but much of the furniture and most of the instruments had disappeared with the military. More were bought and the buildings repaired from the rent paid by the latter, but, wrote a doctor from the former hospital, "there are other changes far more serious ... for which the remedy does not appear:

> "The Chinese houses were destroyed and have not been rebuilt, and as the ground they occupied has been absorbed by the French, Japanese, Russian and German concessions, they probably will not be ... In fact many of those in the French quarter which were not destroyed have been abandoned, either by the order of the French authorities or on account of

> the high rent. The Chinese villages south ... have been occupied by the Indian (Sikh) troops ... patients for the clinics at the hospital have been limited to the school girls from the American Board, our own handful of people ... and the Catholics from the French Concession. This made the number of unbelievers who came very small indeed."

The rebellion had left other legacies as well. There was little night work for Leonora that year, not from fear of the Chinese — nor yet from fear of "the drunken soldier," but "because the specimens of lost humanity, both male and female, who in the wake of the army set up their dens of infamy, drunkenness, and general debauchery ... making it unsafe for a lady to go out at night even to heal the sick."

Another major change that grew out of the war was the treatment of women by men physicians. This practice was still fairly limited, though, and did not seem to be gaining much favour. "In three different cases," wrote a Dr. Benn of the WFMS, "they have confided to me, by way of a compliment, the fact that they first called a French or German doctor and not liking him have come back to me. One woman had undergone a gynaecological operation by a German military surgeon."

Ugly things had been recorded of the German soldiers, but the Methodist doctor reported that one day, a German asked her to see an old lady he had been helping. "An ugly open sore had been dressed as neatly with white bandages as it would have been done in a foreign hospital," she reported. The German had come every day to clean and dress the wound. "Only a common German soldier in a hideous uniform of yellow khaki ... but as I followed him out of that hovel past other hovels where poverty stricken humanity swarmed," one by one the inhabitants related how this unassuming man had helped them. When he saw the hospital, he gave the doctor $4, saying "You <u>must</u> take. Help good work. ... Now I have not (money) but some day give more. Good-bye, I hope you live many years — do good work."

During the sieges, the Emperor, Empress Dowager and their court went into hiding. In September, Prince Ch'ing returned to his palace, protected on all sides by Chinese soldiers. Li Hung-chang returned to Tientsin.

The foreign ministers were formulating a peace document to present to Li and Prince Ch'ing, both of whom were representing the Chinese government in the Emperor's absence. Li, by now old and grey, arrived in Peking October 10, encouraging decisive diplomatic work. On the 16th, he visited the ladies of the legation, after an official call to the American ambassador. The venerable viceroy "seemed to think eating horsemeat ... quite a joke," said

Sarah Conger. "We told him that it was not our food that we remembered with feeling ... but the killing of our people." Li reported that he had sent a private decree to their majesties with regard to punishing the leaders of the uprising, but the foreigners felt they were too insignificant to be considered. Negotiations continued. On December 24, the Joint Note of the nations was handed to Li and Prince Ch'ing. On the 30th, the Chinese government accepted the terms of peace, and on January 16 the document was officially signed.

In March, Leonora watched as the beautiful old walls of Tientsin's Chinese city were levelled by the foreigners, in order to build a boulevard. The Taku forts were destroyed. Alex, itching to leave, must have finally reached a compromise, whereby Leonora would stay and he would go. "I have delayed writing to you on the subject of my furlough as Mrs. King refuses to leave Tientsin at present," he wrote. "I shall leave for home (probably with Mr. Bryson) immediately after our District meetings."[8]

Leonora waited for her patients to trickle back into the city. Few, if any, came in from the countryside. Those who had previously employed the foreigners shut themselves away in their walled compounds. Both city and country were afflicted with former camp-followers, called by one woman missionary, "villains and scum of humanity." Most serious of all, according to the Protestant missionaries, was the change in ownership of the compound buildings. The British buildings having been completely destroyed, the French Catholics extended their holdings, thus presenting a barrier to some Chinese who would not go into, or through, "that French place." Others converted to Catholicism and refused to attend Protestant churches and hospitals.[9]

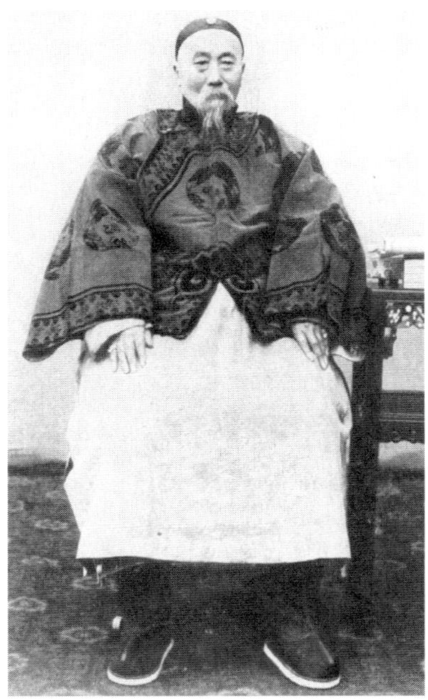

Li Hung-chang

Many of Leonora's patients these days complained of inflamed eyelids, caused by dust, dirt floors and the way "the fire lighters," or wives, had to squat on the floor to push straw into the fireplace. The ashes and smoke made many of these women resort to rubbing their eyes with dirty garments, resulting in worse and worse inflammation, until the eyelashes turned in, scraping the eyeball and in time destroying their sight. Leonora operated on the lids to turn the lashes out and save the eyes. Others came for cataract operations, some of which were successful, but others past all hope of cure.

Even though the Empress Dowager had issued an edict against foot-binding, the practice went on as usual. One little girl, who had been sold into prostitution at age eight, arrived in Tientsin with her feet literally dropping off. Most of the toes were gone, but by careful dressing and cleaning, the rest of the feet were saved. She had begged piteously for the missionaries to keep her, but the most they could do was to make her owners promise not to rebind her feet. The doctor who made out this report noted cynically that the Empress Dowager's edict had been the cause of much rejoicing "at home," not because the practice was so cruel, but because of the expectation of a large Chinese market for American shoes.

In May, the Chinese were presented with an indemnity bill for 450 million taels, or £67 million. The sum was to be paid back by 1940. The Empress Dowager, prompted by Li Hung-chang, signed her country's fortune away on October 27. Li was now partly paralyzed in both legs and could only walk to the negotiating table supported by his servants. Leonora's mentor, the most powerful statesman China had ever known, died on November 7, at age 77. Empress Dowager Tz'u-hsi ordered a shrine to be built in his honour.

How heartbroken Leonora must have been. This great man, a person who had personally protected her, promoted her medical practice and spread Chinese goodwill throughout the world, was gone forever.

Endnotes

1. Fleming, Peter. *The Seige at Peking*. New York: Dorset Press, 1990, pp. 242-243.
2. Benn, Rachel, MD. *Tenth Annual Report of the Woman's Annual Conference of the Methodist Episcopal Church in North China*. Tientsin, China: 1901, pp. 29-35.
3. *Official Minutes of the Ninth Session of the Woman's Annual Conference of the Methodist Episcopal Church in North China*. Tientsin, China: May 24-28, 1901. Boston: The Cushman Press, 1901, pp. 28-29.
4. Stursberg, Peter. *The Golden Hope*. Toronto: United Church Publishing House, 1987, p. 56.
5. Fairbank, John K., ed. *The Missionary Enterprise in China and America*. Cambridge, Mass.: Harvard University Press, 1974, p. 274.
6. Ibid., p. 275.
7. Ibid., p. 279.
8. Council for World Missionary Archives, Day Missions Library, Yale University. London Missionary Society Report Number 63. London: J.D. Liddell, 1901.
9. *Tenth Annual Report of the Woman's Annual Conference of the Methodist Episcopal Church in North China*. Tientsin, China: June 19-21, 1902.

Chapter Twenty-one

The end of an era
1901–1910

Woe to thee, O land, when thy king is a child...
— Ecclesiastes 10:16

Li Hung-chang's death was broadcast around the world, but was felt most keenly by foreigners in Peking and Tientsin, where he had befriended so many of them. Announcement cards were sent to the diplomatic community and to friends such as Leonora and Alex, and permission was given to pay respects at his Peking palace. The ceremonies were phenomenal. In his palace, court after court was filled with visitors, most of whom had brought expensive gifts to express their sympathy and esteem. Flutes wailed and bells tinkled, incense wafted in clouds, and thousands of richly garbed guests partook of great platters of traditional funeral foods. Li's family and his servants would wear coarse white sackcloth for the next two years.

Li's eldest son received condolences in the family's shrine room,[1] where a large portrait of his father hung surrounded by banners and incense burners. Here mourners would kneel on a silken cushion and kowtow three times, striking their heads against the floor. Most of the foreigners would have simply bowed, but it is possible that Leonora and Alex would, this time, have followed Chinese tradition and kowtowed as a final gesture to their great friend. Behind Li's portrait were heavy silken curtains, and beyond that his huge, intricately carved casket, where the rest of his family mourned.

Li Hung-chang's funeral was the most elaborate the foreigners had ever seen. Traditional gifts were exquisite paper flowers placed in equally beautiful replicas of porcelain pots made of papier-maché, all of which would first be displayed, then burned as offerings during the funeral. The ceremonies went on for weeks while shrines and resting pavilions were erected along the funereal route. Finally the procession began. Although most foreigners watched from the wayside,[2] it is likely Leonora would have joined the opulent procession, not walking, but in a richly decorated sedan chair, with umbrella of honour and many outriders, as befitted her rank as a mandarin. Alex would probably have walked beside his wife.

The Empress Dowager had erected a special shrine just outside Peking's city walls. Here, the richly decorated catafalque bearing the remains of China's great Viceroy stopped, while his sons entered the shrine to perform sacred rites. The sons would not be able to hold office nor perform any official duty until two years had passed. His grandson, rather than his eldest son,[3] would bear his royal title. Li Hung-chang was finally laid to rest at one of his palaces in South China.

For Leonora Howard King, Li's death would signal the end of an era. For Imperial China it was the beginning of the end. The Ch'ing dynasty, corrupt and now almost bankrupt, was crumbling. Revolution was in the air. Missionary-educated Dr. Sun Yat-sen, who had entertained dreams of a revolutionary movement in partnership with Li Hung-chang, sat disappointed in Hong Kong, but he would soon make his presence known to Chinese and foreigner alike. It is believed that Leonora's friend Lady Li had passed on a year or so before her husband.[4] After his own death, the rest of his family moved to Canton. The Empress Dowager and Emperor were still in self-imposed exile in Shensi. For the time being, there were few missionaries left in North China.

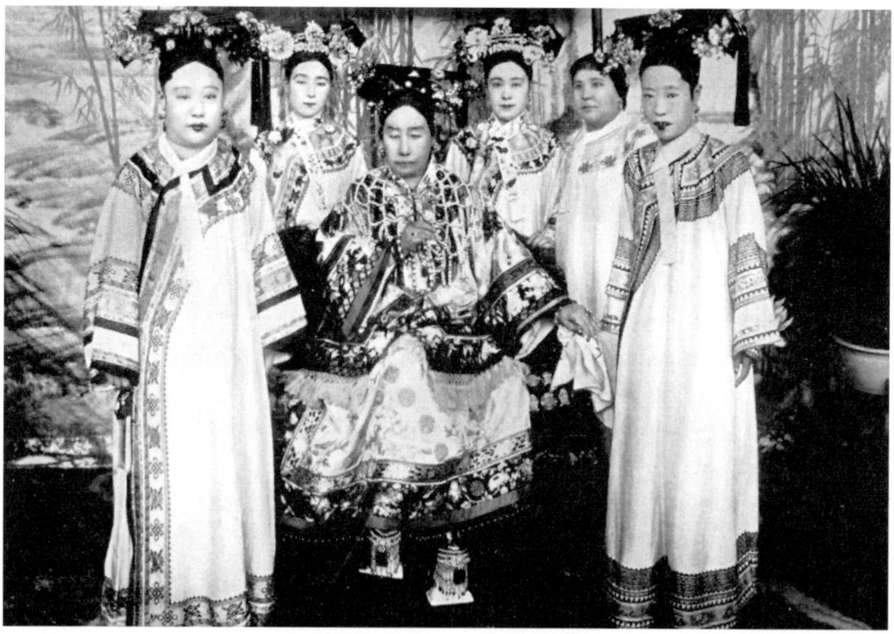

The Empress Dowager and ladies of her court

In August and September, the Empress Dowager shocked traditionalists by banning the "Essay with Eight Legs," which had ensured a livelihood for scholars for centuries. A new Ministry of Education sprang up in Peking. The old imperial university was reinaugurated among crowds of cheering students who welcomed a new scientific era. Tientsin and Shanghai became the centres of a new Westernized movement. Leonora and Alex, who deplored the continuing presence of armed forces in Tientsin, saw a number of military schools erected in their city.

In spring 1901, Alex finally got his wish to return to England and Scotland, where he stayed on furlough from June 19 to October 4, 1902. Leonora herself spent some time in Vienna, where she had previously attended medical conferences. Considering her strong aversion to England, she probably spent time there during the summer months only. She was so attached to China, however, it is likely she returned to Tientsin before Alex had completed his furlough.

In January 1902, North China was abuzz with the news that the Emperor, the Empress and Empress Dowager Tz'u-hsi were returning to court. Preparations for their return had taken hundreds of workmen many months. Because the beautiful Ch'ien Men gates had been burned during the Boxer troubles, the Chinese quickly constructed elaborate towers decorated with royal emblems. Travelling by Belgian and then British trains for the last legs of her journey, she broke tradition by allowing the populace to gaze upon her face. Once ensconced in the Forbidden City, she held an audience with the foreign ministers, and invited the legation ladies back for a more informal visit.

The Throne made sweeping changes. To conservative Chinese, they were appalling. Manchu and Han Chinese could now marry each other; footbinding was illegal; men of the imperial clan could study overseas; and state schools were to be opened for both boys and girls. In 1903, after Leonora and Alex had returned to Tientsin, the Empress Dowager created a Ministry of Commerce. In 1905, she abolished the traditional Confucian-based examinations, which had been held in China since AD 622. The Tsungli Yamen was replaced by the Wai-wu-pu, or Ministry of Foreign Affairs. She ordered that customs, previously run by foreigner Sir Robert Hart, was to be operated by Chinese only.

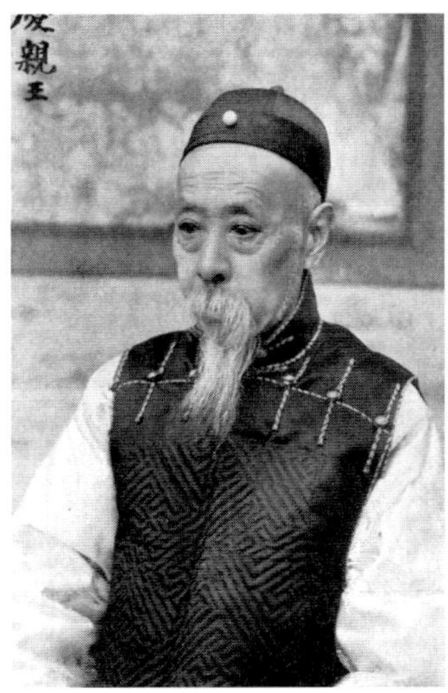

Prince Ch'ing, Premier of China, one of the negotiators in 1900

Most of these reforms emanated from missionary-educated Chinese, who were tired of dynastic corruption. Many had already heard of Dr. Sun Yat-sen's revolutionary manifesto to "Restore China," (to the Chinese), "Establish the Republic," "Equalize Land Ownership" and, most threatening, to "Drive out the Tartars," or Tz'u-hsi and her fellow Manchus. Soon, Shanghai would see the first of many student strikes against corrupt officialdom. Those in the north worried about the presence of Russian armies on the borders of the three eastern provinces.

The missionaries trickled, then flooded back to China, correctly supposing that the mood of reform would prove more friendly to their presence. By 1903, officers and members of the North China Woman's Conference of Leonora's first sponsors, the Methodist Episcopal Church, numbered 31, including six doctors. Hundreds of Chinese returned to her original West Gate dispensary of the Isabella Fisher Hospital, now run by Dr. Emma Martin. "Here," she wrote, "we sometimes have more than we can well manage. Often fifty, seventy-five, or more people are crowded ... in one room, about ten by thirty, furnished only with narrow backless benches, all the light coming in through the paper windows on the north; and containing one small stove the heat of which was perceptible only a few feet away. ... So many cases needing operation ... and we would say, 'Can't you come into our hospital [in the French Concession]; we have nice clean rooms and it will cost you nothing.' And they nearly always say, 'Oh, I would not dare go there. Can't you cure me here?' And they would go away and most ... never come again." The French, being Catholic, were lumped in with the Italians as the most hated and feared of the foreign element, probably due to Chinese superstition about their church rituals.

In 1904, the Russians fought the Japanese on Chinese territory for possession of Manchuria. Empress Dowager Tz'u-hsi suffered a stroke. In Tientsin, Leonora, Alex and their colleagues hosted hundreds of missionaries who had fled Manchuria. Even larger numbers of Chinese and Japanese refugees came to Tientsin to escape the horrors of the war. The number of hospital inpatients had increased over the last year, and many more flooded to the dispensaries.

The Empress Dowager's reforms, including making opium importation illegal, had begun to cut a swath into the trade, and many addicts came for medicine (probably morphine) to help them quit. The general reason was that opium was becoming too expensive. Smallpox was causing more than the usual number of infant deaths. In one town, 300 out of the 700 cases were fatal.[5]

Even though sickness and disease still flourished, life had become a lot easier for Leonora. With better roads, the jinricksha and sedan chair had made way for the horse and carriage. With the proliferation of railroads, she was able to travel in luxury cars, reserved for foreigners and wealthy Chinese. Trips that had previously taken weeks now took mere hours or days. Patients also travelled in these trains, or locally, took street cars that ran straight to her hospital. Many lives were saved as a result of these faster modes of travel.

Medicine in North China had come a long way as well. On the humorous side, there emerged pockets of "surgery fever." Where there was once tremendous resistance to interfering with the physical body, Chinese patients now literally demanded surgery for almost anything. After any successful operation, those who had witnessed the recovery, or even heard about it, fancied that any ailment, from headache to smallpox, could be cured by the knife.

Leonora was now operating three free clinics as well as her hospital. The Isabella Fisher Hospital felt hard done by, both financially and spiritually. "While we have had a busy year," wrote Dr. Emma Martin, "the dispensary work has not been so heavy ... attendance was affected not a little by the three free dispensaries where women are treated within ten minutes walk from us. This also makes a difference in the kind of work we have," she reported, "for the easy cases such as we used to have, never reach us."

In 1908, Leonora opened the Chinese-sponsored Government Medical School for Women, which trained both doctors and nurses. Schoolgirls in uniform, with unbound feet, could be seen walking unattended and unmolested through the streets — a far cry from the pre-Boxer days. Some of the more wealthy actually arrived at school in that new invention, the automobile. The Peking missionaries competed by building the Union Medical College for Women. Instruction was given in Kuan Hua Mandarin, a dialect that "all Chinese from any part of the Empire wish to learn."[6] Students from other parts of China simply attended regular girls' schools to study Kuan Hua until they could understand enough to take the lectures. Apart from attending lectures, Leonora's students learned right on the job.

Cosmetic medicine was on the rise, particularly among the upper classes. Where Leonora had performed dentistry as a matter of course, now there were several dentists in Tientsin who provided the ladies with gold fillings or complete gold teeth. Glass eyes were also catching on. One woman brought her young daughter, who had lost an eye due to an accident, to see if the doctors could "make her beautiful." She asked for a loan of an eye for a week to see if it would fit. When denied the loan, the women left, and hospital staff related that since the young woman was to be married, the woman and her mother wished to borrow the eye until after she had been sent to her mother-in-law. As luck would have it, this mother-in-law was kinder than most, supplying some money to help buy the eye as part of the daughter's trousseau.

In November, Empress Dowager Tz'u-hsi was attacked by dysentery. At the same time the Emperor Kuang-hsu took to his bed. Knowing that they were both dying, Tz'u-Hsi appointed Prince Ch'un II's two year-old son, P'u-i (Pu Yi), emperor successor of China. His father was appointed Regent. On the 14th, the Empress Dowager was well enough to visit the sick Emperor, who in a last gesture of defiance refused to move to the Palace of Peaceful Longevity, or to put on the Robes of Longevity for his deathbed. He died at the Hour of the Cock (between 5 and 7 pm) that very day. The next day Tz'u-hsi arose to discuss the consequences of the Emperor's death with the Grand Council. At lunchtime she apparently had a huge helping of her favourite dish of clotted cream and crabapples. Seized with dysentery again, Tz'u-hsi, the Motherly, Auspicious, Orthodox, Heaven-blessed, Prosperous, All-nourishing, Long-lived, Respectful, Reverent, Worshipful, Illustrious and Exalted, died within a day of her Emperor.[7]

With the Emperor and Empress Dowager dead, the country was thrown into turmoil. People were filled with fear, especially of riot and rebellion. Patients who would otherwise happily have entered Leonora's hospitals stayed huddled in their homes behind blank stone walls. Those who could walk out of the hospital did so, claiming sick relatives and important business at home. The real business at home was preparing for three years' worth of weddings, all to be

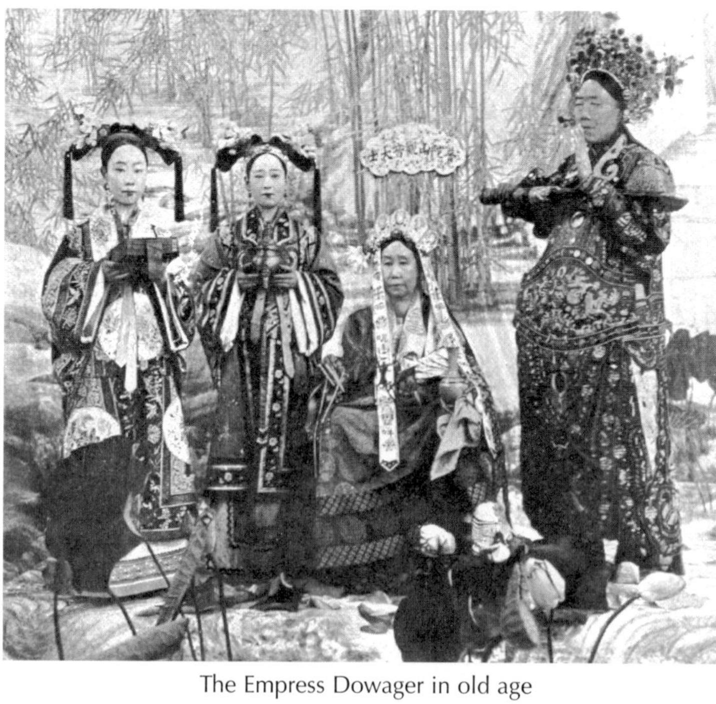

The Empress Dowager in old age

done within the three days of the Emperor's death and the announcement that after three days, everyone was to go into mourning for those next three years.

After those few days, the sick and dying came back, but for months everyone lived under a cloud, both of mourning and uncertainty. Mourning and political turmoil aside, modern medicine marched inexorably forward. Thirty years before, when Leonora had first arrived in China, she had dispensed medicines in whatever shells, cups, bowls, vases, wine-pots and tea-kettles her patients could find. As the foreign community increased and the use of whisky became more common, patients used empty liquor bottles. And now, at the dawn of a new century, patent medicines had made their way across the Pacific. Like the rest of the human race, wrote one doctor, the Chinese tried "the patent medicine first and the doctor last." To counter this trend, Leonora and her colleagues began to dispense their prescription medicines in proper medicine bottles, "although they often bear the stamp of some well known patient [sic] medicine firm."

Clocks, a favourite of Chinese royalty, had ceased to be costly toys of the rich. Many a home now boasted at least one clock that worked, making the task of giving medicines at appropriate times a lot easier. Electrical therapy "for the nerves" had made its way across the ocean as well, and those who had heard of the cure came demanding treatment. Two or three shock treatments seemed to satisfy this latest whim. Much to the medical community's delight, bathing now became very popular. One patient at the Isabella Fisher Hospital was so pleased with the foreign bathtub that she wanted to come back to the hospital every Saturday for a bath and lunch.

But China was still China. After weeks of care and expensive medicine for incipient tuberculosis, one young schoolgirl attributed her recovery entirely to the ingestion of a young boiled owl. When a woman servant who brought in a sick child was told what to feed it, she replied that although she was a church member and broad-minded enough to master the difficulty of an infant diet, the baby's mother was a "heathen" and it would be useless to repeat the doctor's instructions to her. Also, tobacco had found its way into millions of Chinese homes, creating respiratory and cardiac problems that had never been seen in that vast country. In one home of

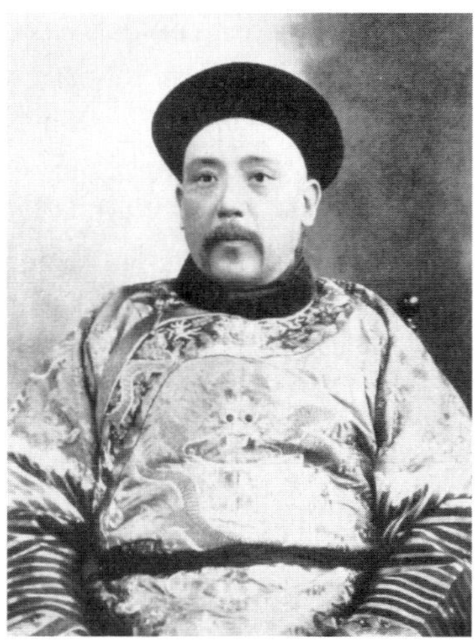

General Yuan Shih-kai

mourning, a doctor found the usual tables with fruits and other food offerings to the dead. Alongside the food were packets of cigarettes.

Leonora's Government Medical School for Women undoubtedly trained nurses as well as doctors. The Chinese students had for a time a depressing existence, having to live in the same premises as their diseased and dying patients. But all the missionary doctors agreed on one thing — the Chinese women were incredibly hard workers, studious and often at their best in cases of emergency.

In progressive Tientsin, sanitary conditions were the best Leonora had ever known. In and near the foreign concessions, most of the new houses (many had been razed during the Boxer Rising) were being built foreign style. The Chinese residents were learning the value of fresh air, water and sunshine. Wages were higher, and families of the coolie classes were better off than they had ever been. Although parents still arranged their children's marriages, it was not now uncommon for young men to be allowed to call on their betrothed. One graduate of the Imperial Medical College (for men) was seen sitting on a sofa with his fiancée, reading from the same book. In former days, these two would not have met each other until the wedding night.

On October 27, 1908, General Yuan Shih-kai, who had been in and out of favour with the ruling court for countless years, was made supreme military and naval commander. Much of China was now being bombarded by revolutionary forces. Shanghai was captured by the revolutionaries on November 4, and a day later a young subaltern named Chiang Kai-shek participated in the capture of the Yamen at Hankow. The Regency appointed Yuan Shih-kai premier of China, a hitherto unknown title, on November 7. Within a month he had dismissed the Regent, formed a cabinet, introduced a new constitution, and made a formal approach to Dr. Sun Yat-sen, leader of a new revolutionary movement, for a peaceful settlement.

Back on November 12, 1866, the boy Sun Yat-sen had been born to a farmer in the village of Choyhung, about 65 kilometres from Canton in the great delta of the West River. He had a normal and happy childhood, worshipping all the right spirits and only rebelling once in school, when he asked the teacher about the meaning of all the characters the children were required to learn by rote. He was severely punished for questioning authority. By age 14, he had never heard the name of Peking, because geography was not taught in Chinese schools. His elder brother Ah Mei had made something of a fortune in Hawaii. It is believed Sun slipped away from his parents to sail to those magic islands.

After clerking for awhile in his brother's general store, he begged Ah Mei to send him to school. The local diocesan college, founded by Bishop Willis of the Church of England, welcomed the boy with open arms. Sun became a devoted assistant at Bible classes and attended both morning and evening prayers. He graduated in 1882, five years after Leonora had arrived in North China. His graduation gift, the second prize in English grammar, was given to him by King Kalakaua. It was a book on missionary life in China and a Bible bound in pigskin. Educated and confident, he returned to China to find a wife.

Although questioning in nature, Sun was not rebellious against the Manchu rulers. This changed radically on the day his boat back to China arrived at the mouth of the Hong Kong harbour. As he told the story, no fewer than three boatloads of corrupt officials came demanding "taxes." Then his fervent Christianity led him to destroy idols and proselytize in his home village. The punishment for this rebellion was death by decapitation or being buried alive in a pit. Only the village's respect for his father saved Sun's life. He was summarily banished to Hong Kong. The Franco-Chinese war in which China lost a tributary country, Annam (Vietnam), to the French was the "critical moment" that determined his life as a revolutionary, determined to save China for the Chinese, and oust the financially and morally bankrupt Manchus. After some months of poverty and inactivity, Sun decided to study medicine in Hong Kong as the first step toward dedicating his life to both the ministry and to a reformed China. In 1892, he received the certificate of proficiency in medicine and surgery — the highest degree available at the time.

Sun practised in South China for awhile, then moved north to Tientsin. It is believed that he wanted to study at Dr. Mackenzie's medical college, supplied and supported by Li Hung-chang. He and his colleague Lu Ho-tung had prepared a study on the deplorable social and political situation existing at the time, and hoped that Li would join him in reforming China. Li did not seem to have read the paper, although it was published in serial form in a Shanghai newspaper the following year.

Back in Hong Kong, Sun Yat-sen inaugurated a new chapter of the Hsing Chung Hui (Revive China Society), a secret revolutionary society that had begun some years before in Macao. A ritual was introduced and all members had to swear allegiance on the Bible. Along with Shanghai resident and prominent Methodist Soong Yao-ju, whose daughter Sun would later marry, he made plans for a revolutionary offensive against Canton as a first step toward revolutionizing the entire country. On September 9, 1895, the day chosen for the insurrection, Sun received a message that 600 pistols would be two days late. Then it was learned that a traitor had infiltrated the secret society. The plans revealed, Sun and his fellow revolutionaries had to retire. He fled to Kobe, Japan, where he cut off his queue.

Sun Yat-sen spent the next year travelling through North America, spreading his gospel of revolution through churches, universities and public gatherings. He was followed by detectives wherever he went. He often attempted to elude them by masquerading as a Japanese. He sailed for London on September 23, 1896. The Chinese minister in Washington, however, had cabled the British asking for his immediate extradition. He was imprisoned in the Chinese legation for a week before a British friend, Dr. Cantlie, finally received a plea for help that he had smuggled out of the building. When Scotland Yard would do nothing, claiming it was a diplomatic issue, Dr. Cantlie hired a firm of detectives, then went to the *Times* office and made a statement, which remained unpublished until after Sun's release. Finally the doctor approached a *Globe* correspondent and they pinned up posters reading "CHINESE REVOLUTIONARY KIDNAPPED IN LONDON." Sun was released on October 23, 12 days after his arrest, and the world was alerted to his cause.

After years of exile in Europe, Japan, Hawaii and Hong Kong, Sun returned to China in 1912, to be made provisional president of a new Chinese Republic. He re-formed his revolutionaries into the more respectable National Peoples' Party, or Kuomintang.

Endnotes

1. Conger, Sarah Pike. *Letters from China*. Chicago: A.C. McClurg & Co., 1910, pp. 213-215.
2. Ibid., pp. 213-215.
3. It is not known why the grandson, rather than the sons, would bear the title.
4. The date of Lady Li's death is unknown to the author.
5. *North China Woman's Conference of the Methodist Episcopal Church*. Peking, May 11th to 14th, 1904. Shanghai and Foochow, China: Lacy & Wilson Methodist Publishing House, 1904, pp. 28-33.
6. *Minutes of the Seventeenth Session of the North China Woman's Conference of the Methodist Episcopal Church*. Peking, September 29th to October 4th, 1909. Shanghai and Foochow, China: Methodist Publishing House, 1909, pp. 51-60.
7. Warner, Marina. *The Dragon Empress: The Life and Times of Tz'u-hsi, 1835-1908, Empress Dowager of China*. London: Cardinal, 1974, pp. 259-260.

Chapter Twenty-two

A place to rest
1925

"I have been a stranger in a strange land ... "
— Exodus 2:22

While Leonora and Alex had been away on furlough, the Pei Ho River, "the monster," had begun to be tamed through a massive engineering effort that contained the river and allowed a boulevard to be built in Tientsin's European district. Now, wide open spaces invited the occasional fresh breeze. Even the narrow, ever-crowded streets in the Chinese district had been paved, if not widened. At nighttime thousands of little shops sparkled like precious jewels, their canopies bedecked with strings of real electric lights. In the midst of all this modernization, babies still cried and were comforted, meals were peddled to passers-by, and China went on.

In the next few years, Leonora's medical school produced well-trained Chinese doctors — all women. Bright young nurses-in-training strove to wear the crisp blue cap and uniform — white was the colour of mourning — of the graduate. The work never lacked variety. One day an old lady of 70 was found with four big needles stuck in her abdomen. There was a great crowd of people standing around to see what the foreign doctors could do and, wrote one medical woman, "our first impulse was to leave the case at once," but they pulled the needles out and made her as comfortable as possible. The old woman developed peritonitis afterward, but recovered remarkably well. The Western doctors had heard of acupuncture before, but had never actually dealt with it.

The practice of foot-binding, although outlawed by the late Empress Dowager, continued. A WFMS report said "anyone who has never seen a bound foot with the bandages recently removed cannot realize the awfulness of this custom till they see the pink quivering mass of shapeless flesh." One day a little girl was carried in. She was running an open sore from a broken bone in her foot. After the doctors had dressed the foot as comfortably as possible, the old women who had brought her in began replacing the original foot-bandage, binding it as tightly as possible. The doctors protested vehemently, but to no avail.

In emergencies, Leonora was often called upon to help Dr. Emma Martin, the newest doctor at the Isabella Fisher Hospital. Between crises, they must have shared a good laugh at the following story: "One day a woman came in and greeted my assistant as an old friend," wrote Dr. Martin. [She] said: 'Oh! we have a new doctor. What is her name?' We told her and asked what was the matter, and she said the toothache." It seemed strange, related the doctor, to have anyone speak so cheerfully about the toothache, and she enquired more minutely about the problem. "In the meantime she took from the depths of her garment a small package around which was wrapped carefully in a dirty little rag, and to my surprise she showed me the teeth which had been extracted in previous years. She laughed and said, 'Dr. Gloss pulled these two, and Dr. Barrow this one, and Dr. Benn this, and Dr. Stevenson these.'" Emma Martin extracted the tooth, "for which she thanked me heartily, and laughed in glee as she put this curious souvenir with the others."

In 1909, North China was swept by smallpox, diphtheria and scarlet fever. In 1910, the pneumonic plague spread its deadly tentacles down from Manchuria. Cases of plague were reported daily in Peking, and the medical field experienced considerable alarm. To protect themselves, their students and their existing patients, hospitals closed the inpatient departments. Happily, the rumours of death were overblown, and there had actually been very few cases of real plague. Tientsin, as the port to Peking, was carefully guarded by a large staff of physicians and police officers, who kept the city in quarantine for a time. Rail travel was only allowed by special permission. In other parts of China, people would never isolate themselves in cases of disease, but in large part thanks to Leonora, the populace of Tientsin had "been educated up to foreign medicine and seldom call us [the doctors] too late."

There were now two medical colleges in Tientsin — Leonora's and an institution for male students. The Chinese graduates and the missionary doctors shared pleasant professional relations. Just before the child Emperor, Pu Yi, was officially deposed in 1912, Leonora, her students and graduates alike made thousands of first aid packages for the newly arrived Red Cross Society. The work continued for weeks in the expectation of an attack on Peking by southern revolutionaries.

Sun Yat-sen's attempts at revolution, while they did not close her hospitals, changed the character of medical missionary work considerably. A much poorer class of patient was now arriving at the Isabella Fisher Hospital, and treatment was expected to be free. Leonora's own work would not have changed substantially, because her government hospitals never charged fees, relying, instead, on donations from the rich and powerful, many of whom had fled Peking and were renting properties in the foreign concessions. Her students became invaluable, not only filling prescriptions and explaining dosages in a way that could be better accepted by the Chinese mind, but giving lectures on the care and feeding of infants, the use of soap and water, fresh air, clean drinking water and proper food.

In Peking, fearful of civil war, people started demanding hospital rooms at almost any price, rather than be attacked in their own homes. For weeks one hospital was besieged daily by men who wanted to engage a room for a relative. "One, two, sometimes three rooms they demanded," wrote one woman doctor, "but when it came to the important question of the illness ... we discovered

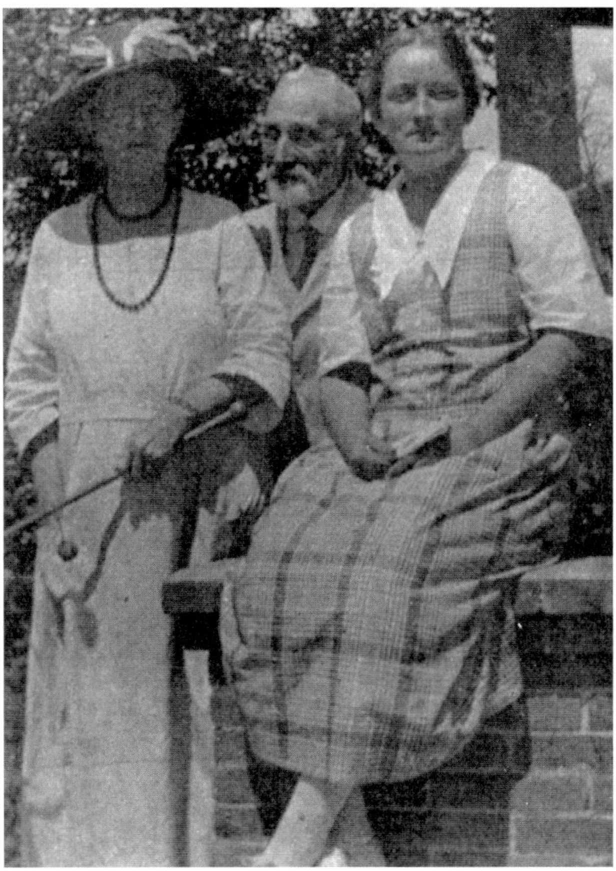

On the right is Agnes Clarke, adopted daughter

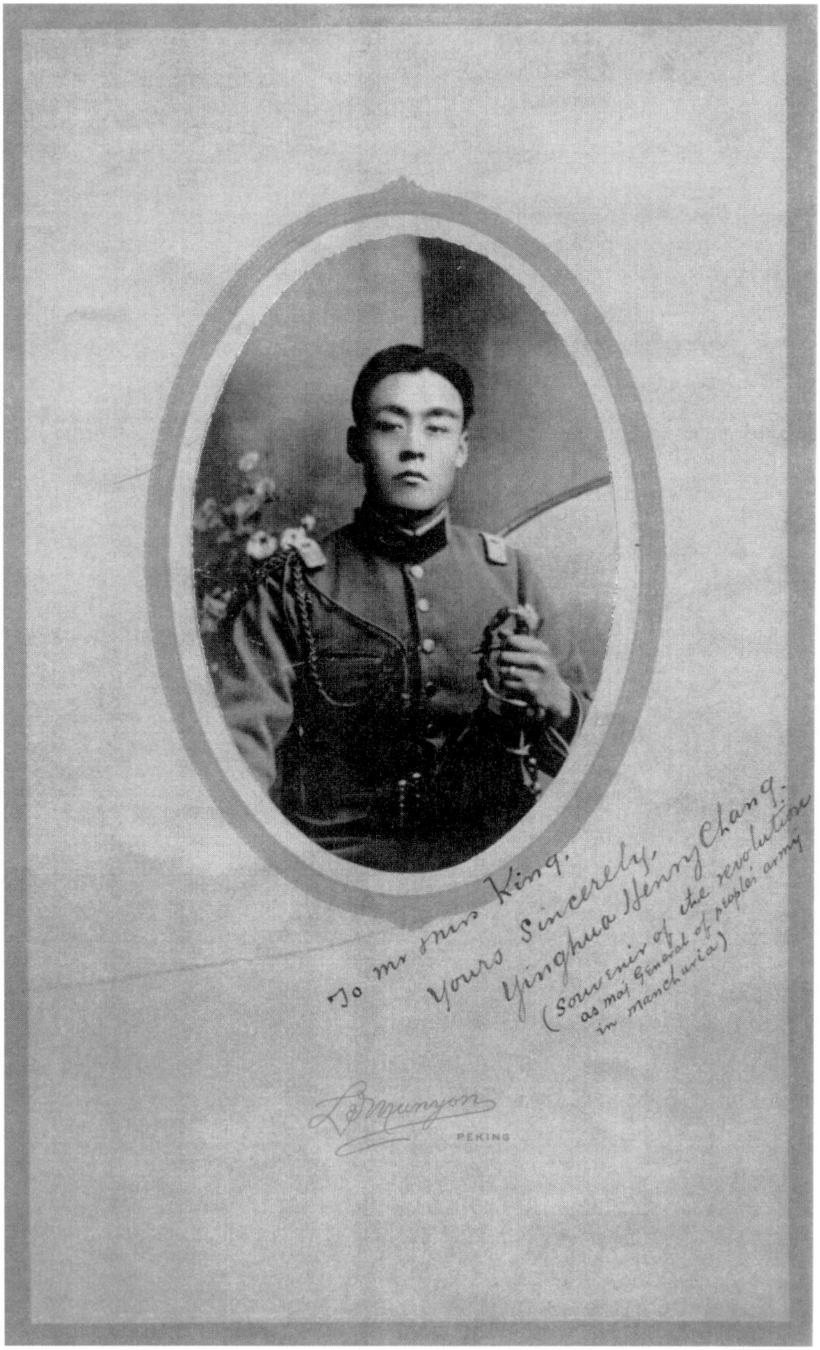

Notes from a friend

that the lady was not ill at all. They simply wanted to rent the rooms." The hospitals began selecting cases that would be in the greatest danger until all the wards were full, and then told the others that in case of an attack on Peking, they would allow space on the floors. They would agree to take a patient, but when she arrived, it was found that this meant taking the patient, several children, a servant or two and a great pile of boxes. Great offence was taken when admission for all but the patient was refused on the ground that the hospital must be kept for the sick.

After the abdication of the Manchu Emperor, Leonora and her colleagues felt the great strain that everyone had undergone would be lifted, but this was not to be. Directly on the heels of the celebration of the new republic came unmanageable soldiers after the spoils of war. According to ancient Chinese custom, after a war had ended the soldiers would be permitted to loot as a reward for bravery. This was a dark page in the history of the republic, wrote one missionary doctor, "but after a few decapitations and the help of foreign soldiers, peace was once more restored." Many Chinese women and children were left homeless.

Some time during this period Leonora and Alex adopted Agnes Clarke, the daughter of two British missionaries who had been killed during a disturbance. Little is known of Agnes, except that she kept her own name and on reaching the age of majority, she returned to her English home, then went back to China as a missionary. It is believed that she, like her parents, was also killed during an anti-foreign demonstration.

In January 1913, Leonora and more than 70 physicians from all parts of China attended the five-day Triennial Conference of the Medical Missionary Association in Peking. One of the conference's most important results was the issuing of a "Policy of Medical Mission Work," part of which read: "Amongst the most pressing needs of medical missions is the further development of work amongst women and children. We therefore recommend that such work be extended to as many centres as possible."

On March 27 and 28, 1915, the WFMS rejoiced at the opening of a brand new Isabella Fisher Hospital. It is certain that Leonora and Alex would have attended, as did all the provincial officials who lived in Tientsin, with the exception of the governor, who was in mourning, but sent his representative, the commissioner of foreign affairs. Chinese friends were pleased to give "gold $100" to name a room for a loved one. The doctors consulted among themselves and named one room in honour of Leonora, as the first WFMS physician in Tientsin.

In 1917, floods nearly swept the city off the map, but the solid foreign structures withstood the assault. Leonora and Alex both officially retired, at the

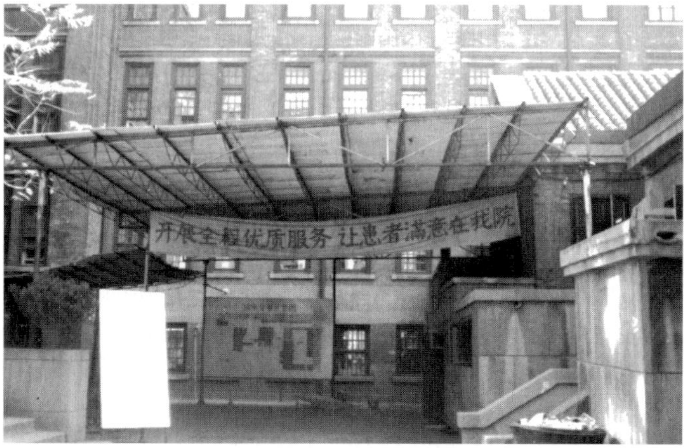

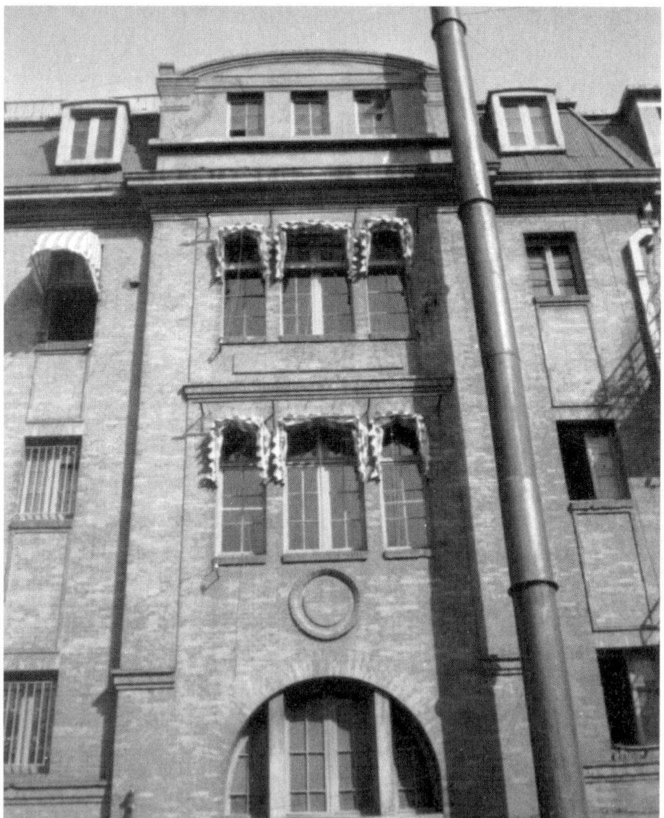

Government Hospital for Women and Children, Tientsin
(Above and below)

respective ages of 66 and 67, but according to WFMS records they continued to give their service of healing and love. During this time the British minister Sir Robert MacLeay visited Tientsin to open a new block of the Mackenzie Memorial Hospital, named for Leonora's now-deceased colleague Dr. Mackenzie, or "Ma Taifu." Taku Road was gay with flags, motorcars, brass bands and fashionable people, Chinese and foreign alike. His Excellency Sir Robert and Lady MacLeay shared the platform with the Civil Governor, the Commissioner of Foreign Affairs, and numerous distinguished guests, including Dr. C.P. Wang, general secretary of the YMCA and of course, Alex and Leonora. A troop of Chinese Boy Scouts, who had recently walked from Tientsin to Peking,* formed at the entrance and smartly saluted the visitors on arrival.

In his speech the British minister stressed: "This hospital is primarily intended for the poorer classes of Chinese. The development of industralism [sic], the increased use of machinery, and the dangers of our streets all add to the risk of life, especially among the working classes ... the number of outpatients treated last year was 38,538, an increase of 867 over ... the preceding year." He ended with a strong plea for funds to further modernize Ma Taifu's hospital.

General Wang Cheng-pin, civil governor of Chihli, then spoke in the same vein, adding: "Personally, I will welcome any movement in secure [sic] funds for this hospital, and will do my best. Thirty years ago foreign medicine in China was not well appreciated and its efficacy was not well known, but now it is different. As a military man, I know of the work of doctors on the battlefield, where they have gone about their labour of love under most trying conditions amid great hazards and discomforts. We should do our very best to acknowledge their great services both in time of war and peace."

British missionary Dr. Stuckey concluded the speeches, saying "The name we have met to honour today is that of Dr. Mackinzie [sic]. He is unfortunately no longer with us. But we rejoice to have with us today Dr. Mackenzie's lady colleague, Dr. King, who assisted him in attendance on Lady Li. It is my pleasure, in behalf of the hospital committee, to ask her to present to Sir Ronald Macleay a silver key with which to open the new building." After Dr. Stuckey's address had been translated into Chinese by Dr. Wang, Leonora, *Ke ye-da tai-tai*, handed the British minister the key. "Sir Ronald, in accepting it, said he felt it all the greater honour to receive the key from the hands of such a distinguished medical lady, whose name was linked with charity and kindness of heart."[1]

*The newspaper reporter probably meant from Peking to Tientsin.

The year 1921 brought another terrible famine, which drew heavily on medical resources during the long cold winter. Relief services were given to tens of thousands of refugees who were housed in tent camps in Tientsin. Many of these refugees had never before been exposed to modern medicine and hundreds of obstetrical cases were taken into the warmth of the Western hospitals, given care never before dreamed of, and sent away with clean warm clothing.

But the Tientsin government was tightening its belt. In 1922, in response to Leonora's request for $1,200 to keep the Government Hospital for Women and Children open, the bureaucrats replied that the hospital was a private business and should not use government subsidies. In any case, they said, the government was running on a deficit. Leonora promptly replied that because she received no salary, it could not be a private business. She also sent a petition asking for more women doctors. "The clinic is losing money," read one of her pleas for help. "You can help thousands of people every year. It is money well-spent. Please reverse your decision."

Then Leonora really went to work, inviting friends in high places for a social gathering at her home. She explained that the $1,200 was, in fact, funding for an entire year — "the average needed monthly, in fact, is only $100, including paying for Chinese doctors and nurses, and of course cleaning staff."[2] It is not known if she received her funding, but a negative answer may very well have affected her decision to return to Canada.

In 1923, Leonora and Alex spent the summer in Ontario with her brother Eugene and his wife Eliza Ann. Cousin Hilliard and his wife Stella, nephews Stanley, Charles and Clarence, their wives Janet, Margaret and Gertrude, great nieces Dorothy and Geraldine and great nephew George all got together at Eugene's farm in Athens for family photographs. During her visit, Leonora gave a brief address on the lawn at the Athens United Church, meeting and greeting a few old friends and chatting with "the children" of those she had known in her girlhood. A Leeds county newspaper reported: "At that time, Dr. Howard-King [sic] was 72 years of age, but appeared 20 years or so younger. She planned to return to China with her husband, and, after settling their financial matters there, they would return to Leeds county and spend the remainder of their lives amongst their friends and relatives."[3] Tall and imposing, the former shy

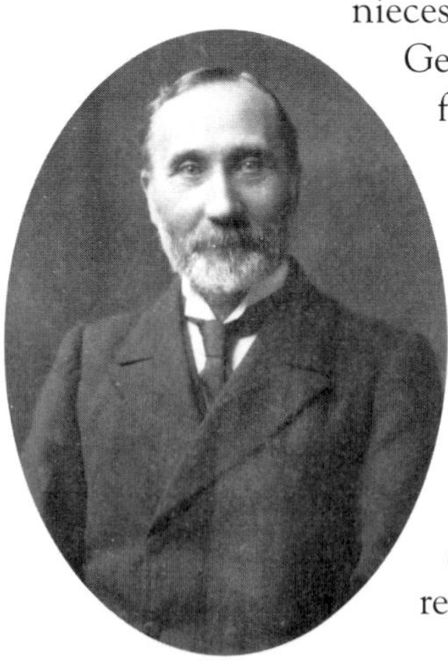
Alex in Scotland, 1923

country girl spoke to her audiences "with the voice of authority," but with the children she was as gentle and loving as ever.[4]

On November 5, deposed Emperor Pu Yi was forced to leave the Forbidden City. He moved to Tientsin and was now a "guest" in the Japanese concession, just about a mile from Leonora and Alex's city residence.

On January 31, 1924, Leonora wrote to her nephew Clarence: "We miss you all very much. Wish often that you could come to our home, just as you did to your dad's. Wouldn't it be fine? This week I gave a large lunch party and wished my own people were there. Such reflections are of no use. I wished to talk over family and some business matters (during the visit to Canada) but in the hurry did not do so ... Love to all, Aunt Leonore [sic]."

Sun Yat-sen died of liver cancer on March 12, 1925. His last words were said to be "*Ho* … *Ho* … *Ping, fan-dao, chiu* … *chiu* … *chung-kuo*" — "Peace ... struggle ... save China."

On May 30, some pro-union workers at Shanghai Cotton Mill Number Two were fired by their Japanese managers. In the ugly strike that followed, a Japanese worker murdered a young Chinese employee. Within the hour, Shanghai students who supported the union moved urgently from factory to factory, spreading word of the young man's martyrdom.

By midday, a huge crowd was milling in front of a department store on Nanking Road. At precisely 12:15 pm a gun went off. At this signal, thousands of multicoloured pamphlets fluttered through the air like so much confetti. The pamphlets were grasped by eager, searching hands and read hungrily. Mingling with the crowd, the organizers brandished bright red flags, home-made signs and gigantic banners that snapped like firecrackers in the searing Shanghai breeze. More students, perched on steps, lamp-posts, any vantage-point, exhorted the crowd to claim their rights as Chinese citizens and protest against foreign exploitation. The crowd, now 5,000 strong, marched eight abreast to the local police station.

The British police, ruddy and moist under their pith helmets, were not quite sure what to do. One officer, in an attempt to placate the marchers, suggested they demonstrate in the Chinese part of the city — this was foreign concession land. The students hotly refused, asserting that this was Chinese land and they had more right to be there than the British. The workers, encouraged, joined in with shouts and jeers, but the police stood their ground in the broiling sun, well-oiled boots planted firmly on the steps. Finally a message, or "chit," was sent to the police inspector, who was attempting to break 90 on the immaculate greens of the Bund's beautiful golf course. Annoyed at the interruption, he curtly sent an order for his staff to open fire. Eleven Chinese were killed that day. Within the week, fierce anti-British demonstrations had broken out in 28 Chinese cities.*

To make matters worse there was another devastating famine in Chihli province. It was inevitable that dysentery, cholera, malarial outbreaks and typhoid would march bleakly beside the refugees who poured into the cities. Although many patrons among the wealthier classes had sought seclusion during the political troubles, Chinese medical staff in Tientsin remained calm and reasonable, but by no means passive. Rather than seek seclusion as well, they proceeded to "march in uniform, ready for service."

After she had returned from Canada, the Tientsin officials had refused to let Leonora practise medicine. Whether they had cited her retirement of 1916 or the new "China for the Chinese" philosophy is unknown. Although Leonora had taken the rejection well, the government's decision had still been a bitter blow. In some sort of recompense she had been paraded around, opening this, cutting the ribbon at that, remembering *not* to bow to remaining royalty. Young Chinese "moderns" now bobbed their hair, danced the Charleston, and drank English gin. Everyone smoked cigarettes. Even his majesty, deposed Emperor "Henry" Pu Yi, danced the Tango in the Astor hotel's ballroom. The Charleston, with its frenzied kicks, and the Tango, with its sensual dips, were enough to make the Empress Dowager turn over in her grave. It was time to go home to Canada.

Leonora had the 'flu. How odd that after all those years of malaria, all those years of exposure to every deadly disease known to medicine, she would contract such a common virus. A rueful smile might have given her plain, rather severe fact the soft radiance that had charmed the Chinese, from highest official to the poorest peasant.

June billowed in with a fresh tang of sea air that mingled with the voluptuous scent of Petaiho's summer blossoms. Already the missionary resort community was bright with sweet peas, triumphant morning glory and huge white vining clematis. Leonora's own garden danced with a riot of cosmos blossoms. The doctor had come to say goodbye for the last time to the lovely bungalow she and Alex had built back in 1895. This charming summer residence was crowned with a gently curving Chinese roof made of warm red tiles. Neat brickwork and smooth whitewashed pillars supported a broad shady verandah, dotted here and there with comfortable cane chairs and small bamboo tables. Six steps led down to the quiet lawns of Leonora's garden. The house itself was

*Interview with former Shanghai factory worker, BBC television presentation "China Rising," Arts and Entertainment Network, 1994.

light, airy and spacious, a country haven that blended the best of East and West. The walls of the servants' quarters were inlaid with large, multi-coloured stones, reminiscent of the stone homesteads one found back in Ontario's small neat towns.

Leonora might have continued to smile at the thought that most "foreigners," even that woman-hating cynic, Somerset Maugham, thought the missionaries took extended vacations by the sea because they were lazy. Old China Hands, which she now most definitely was, knew better. When the mission boards at home had objected to this "annual leave," those in the field had responded tartly that if the Lord's work were to continue, they must either have an healthful escape-hatch, or they would invoice for funeral expenses![5] The tranquil resort of Peitaiho had been created as a sanitarium for missionaries who contracted any of the dozens of illnesses that threatened their daily work.

Who knows what sadness must have filled her as she packed her prized possessions — here was a tea set of ebony with silver dragons, given to her by Lady Li in bygone years — there the bronze plaque, reading: "A doctor is interested in curing people, not in money" that had been presented by the Viceroy when the Isabella Fisher Hospital had first opened. Exquisite vases were packed along with intricately carved cups and bowls, and a chain-mesh belt made out of pure silver went into her personal luggage. Leonora's jewellery, including a beautiful

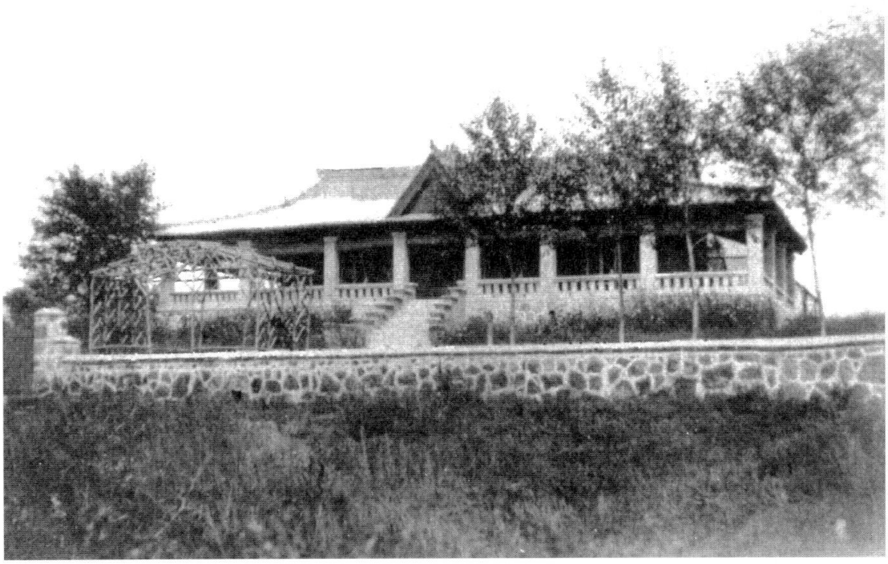

A place to rest

garnet brooch, a gold pendant inlaid with precious stones, and delicate silver-and-turquoise earrings would remind her of the China she had loved and served for 47 years. Finally a picture of Leonora, Alex and their adopted daughter Agnes Clarke was slipped into a roomy handbag.*

It would be nice to think that Leonora, always a proponent of fresh air, fought this latest virus by asking her servants to place her bed on the wide verandah overlooking the sea. Perhaps she saw a gleaming black cormorant circling over the vast sunlit ocean. Is that you, old friend Li? The Chinese, with their eternal, impossible lists of gods and souls and after-lives, could be practically anything in the spirit world.

A temple gong might have chimed in the distance. Dragons danced in the wild white clouds that had puffed up in the brilliant blue morning. Dragons with forked tails. Dragons with golden scales. Big dragons chased little dragons across the soft bright sky, smoke whooshing from their wide flared nostrils. China had been Leonora's personal dragon, the wondrous, ageless dragon that the foreigners had wanted to slay. But they would never succeed.

THE END

Endnotes

1. Howard Family Collection. "Ma Taifu's Hospital - Visit of the British Minister - A Chance for Wealthy Donors -The Old Buildings Falling in," *North China Daily Mail.* Date unknown.
2. Personal papers obtained from Miss Geraldine Howard.
3. Howard Family Collection. Towriss, Louise. "A Distinguished Daughter of Leeds County." June 30, 1935.
4. Personal communication with Miss Geraldine Howard, Toronto.
5. Hunter, Jane. *The Gospel of Gentility - American Women Missionaries in Turn-of-the-Century.* New Haven: Yale University Press, 1984. p. 146.

*These items were brought back to Canada and remain in the family.

Epilogue

I have fought the good fight, I have finished my course, I have kept the faith.
— Timothy 4:7

Leonora Howard King died of a virus on June 30, 1925. Here is her obituary:

"News has been received of the death of Mrs. Leonora Howard King, of Tientsin, China, wife of the Rev. Alexander King of the London Missionary Society.

"Mrs. King came to China forty-seven years ago, from Canada, the country of her birth, and served as a medical missionary in charge of the Isabella Fisher Hospital, Taku Road, founded by the Methodist Episcopal Mission. At the last annual meeting of the Mackenzie Memorial (London Mission) Hospital, Taku Road, when Mr. and Mrs. King were both present, reference was made to the fact that Mrs. King became a colleague of Dr. Mackenzie and to the happy accident, if it could be called an accident, of her introduction into the family of the Viceroy Li Hung-chang, whose wife she attended with successful results, thus winning the great Viceroy's lifelong interest in and support of Western medicine and of the London Mission Hospital. Mrs. King left the Methodist Episcopal Mission on her marriage to Mr. Alexander King and ultimately carried on a women's hospital and dispensary of her own, together with her own practice, chiefly among the Chinese. Her work was quite voluntary and free, given out of the goodness of her heart, and was independent of the Mission of which she was a member by marriage. Whether it were foreigner or

> Chinese, rich or poor, distinguished or lowly, Dr. King gave her skill and time to those who demanded it, never making any professional charges, but devoting herself mainly to attendance on Chinese women, with a degree of tireless activity that caused her friends to marvel. Last year Mr. and Mrs. King made a trip to Canada — Mrs. King's second visit home in forty-seven years. Mr. King himself has only been home about twice in his long residence in China.
>
> Speaking of Mrs. King's death the *North China Daily Mail* says: "At this time of political disturbances and international quarrels it seems as if we were all reproached when we think of her quiet, unostentatious life, the nobility and gentleness of her medical work, the lifelong voluntary sacrifice of self for the benefit of others."[1]

Another newspaper memorial reads:

> "The career of Dr. Leonora Annette [sic] Howard King, who has just died in far-off and strife-torn China, furnishes an illustration of what may be accomplished by Canadian girls and should serve as an inspiration to others who may be facing life's trials and uncertainties ... .
>
> "Leonora Howard had courage as well as determination ... we may imagine that at the outset her labors were attended by difficulties which might well have appeared insuperable to men and women of less faith and strength of character ... .
>
> "It was a far cry from a Leeds county [word missing] to favoritism at an Oriental court. Not every woman would have been able to accomplish the feat. But Dr. Howard had peculiar powers which enabled her to overcome all the obstacles which beset her path and in the hour of her death, at an advanced age, it is fitting that tribute should be paid to her by the people of her native shire and that her name should be listed among those Leeds country men and women who have contributed, and contributed nobly, to the betterment of humanity."[2]

Leonora's story fell into obscurity with the passage of time. Her letters home were lost sometime in the 1960s. If she kept a diary, it has never surfaced. Had it not been for the tremendous cooperation of her great-nieces and great-nephew, I might have given up chasing this interesting ghost long ago. As luck would have it, Alex was a prodigious correspondent and also recording secretary of the Peking District Missionary Society. With Alex's unwitting help, I hope I have painted a picture, with some predictable gaps, of almost 50 years of this extraordinary woman's life. This book was compiled using Leonora's and other reports to the Woman's Foreign Missionary Society, many other contemporary missionary references, and hundreds of Alex's letters as recording secretary. Leonora was "humanized," regarding her personality, her taste in clothing, jewellery, and her love of China with the great help of the Howard family, some of whom had met Leonora, and most of whom remembered Alex.

Alex King outlived his wife by another 14 years. On returning from Canada to China to bury Leonora, he found that their "financial manager" had absconded with most of their considerable fortune. According to London Missionary Society records, two years later Alex settled in Canada, near Leonora's relatives in Athens, Ontario. Alex finally retired to Boscombe, England, where he died at age 88 on January 20, 1939.

Eugene Howard also outlived his sister Leonora. He died near Athens, in 1936. He was also 88.

The Memorial Temple of Tseng Kuo-fan is now part of San Tiao Shi High School at 16 North Road of the South Canal, Tianjin, China. Although two original buildings are still standing, they are dilapidated.

Leonora's Government Hospital for Women and Children, Dagu (Taku) Road, Tianjin, is now the Ophthalmologist Hospital of Tianjin.

Her medical and nursing school at 182 Ansan road continues as the Tianjin Nursing School.

The French Legation building on Chengde Road, Tianjin, became the Public Benefit Bureau. It is now the Library for Children.

The French Legation building on Northern Jeifang Road became the Public Benefit Bureau, and is now the Tianjin Food Bureau.

The British Legation buildings were destroyed in the Boxer Rebellion. The former location houses the current municipal government.

The Astor Hotel, after years of neglect, has been restored to its former splendour through a joint venture between the City of Tianjin and a Hong Kong consortium.

The former residence and gravesite of Li Hung-chang have been totally destroyed. There are several statues of him in the Tianjin History Museum, Guanghua Road, Hexi District.

Leonora Howard King's home and gravesite cannot be found. It is believed that these sites were destroyed during Communist/Nationalist disturbances.

Endnotes

1. *New Outlook* (August 12, 1925), p. 25.
2. Newspaper clipping supplied by the Howard family. Publication unknown.

Equivalent spellings and terminology

Colonial/Wade-Giles System	Pinyin/Modern-day terminology
Boxer Rebellion/Uprising	Boxer Rising/Boxer Incident
Canton/Kwangchow	Guangzhou
Chiang Kai-shek	Jiang Jieshi
Chihli Province	Zhili
Ch'ing Dynasty	Qing Dynasty
Compradore	Go-between
Formosa	Taiwan
Huang Ho (Yellow River)	Huang He
Kuomintang/KMT/Nationalists	Guomindang
Li Hung-chang	Li Hongzhang
Nanking	Nanjing
Pei Ho (River)	Hei He
Peitaho	Beidahe
Peking	Beijing
Shantung Province	Shandong
Sun Yat-sen	Sun Zhongshan
The Son of Heaven	The Emperor
The Middle Kingdom	China
Tientsin	Tianjin
Tientsin Massacre	Tianjin Incident
Tsungli Yamen	Government Foreign Office
Tz'u-hsi/Empress Dowager	Ci Xi
Vietnam/Annam	Dong Jing
Yamen	Government meeting hall

Selected reading

Austin, Alvyn J. *Saving China - Canadian Missionaries in the Middle Kingdom, 1888-1959*. Toronto: University of Toronto Press, 1986.

Barrett, David B., ed. *World Christian Encyclopedia*. Nairobi: Oxford University Press, 1982.

Bird, Isabella. *The Yangtze Valley and Beyond*. London: Virago Press Edition, 1985.

Buck, Pearl S. *China As I See It*. New York: John Day Company, 1970.

Chen, Stephen and Robert Payne. *Sun Yat-sen: A Portrait*. New York: John Day Company, 1946.

Conger, Sarah Pike. *Letters from China*. Chicago: A.C. McClurg & Co., 1910.

Cross, F.L. and E.A. Livingstone, eds. *Oxford Dictionary of the Christian Church*. 2nd edition. Oxford: Oxford University Press, 1983.

Fairbank, John K., ed. *The Missionary Enterprise in China and America*. Cambridge, Mass.: Harvard University Press, 1974.

Fleming, Pater. *The Siege at Peking*. New York: Dorset Press, 1990.

Frazer Smith, James, Reverend, MD, CM. *Life's Waking Part*. Toronto: Thomas Nelson and Sons, Limited, 1937.

Graves, R.H., D.D. *Forty Years in China or China in Transition*. Baltimore, Maryland: R.H. Woodward Company, 1895.

Hacker, Carlotta. *The Indomitable Lady Doctors*. Federation of Medical Women of Canada. Toronto: Clark & Irwin & Company Inc., 1974.

Hunter, Jane. *The Gospel of Gentility - American Women Missionaries in Turn-of-the-Century China*. New Haven: Yale University Press, 1984.

Kwang-Ching Liu, ed. *American Missionaries in China*. Cambridge, Mass.: East Asian Research Center, Harvard University Press, 1970.

Latourette, K.S. *A History of Christian Missions in China*. London: Society for Promoting Christian Knowledge, 1929.

Liu Jiantang and Tian Yutang, eds. *Astor Hotel Sightseeing Over a Century. Tianjin*, People's Republic of China: Tianjin People's Publishing House, 1993.

Maugham, W. Somerset. *On a Chinese Screen*. Oxford: Oxford University Press, 1922.

McCutcheon, Marc. *Everyday Life in the 1800s*. Cincinnati, Ohio: Writer's Digest Books, 1993.

Mericka, Vaclav. *Orders and Decorations*. Trans. Dermot Morrah, ed. London: Paul Hamlyn Ltd., 1967.

Morrison, G.E. (Chinese). *An Australian in China*. Sydney, Australia: Angus and Robertson Pty. Ltd., 1972.

Purcell, Victor. *The Boxer Uprising*. Cambridge: Cambridge University Press, 1963.

Smith, Arthur H. *The Uplift of China*. New York: Forward Mission Study Courses. Young People's Missionary Movement, 1907.

Stursberg, Peter. *The Golden Hope*. Toronto: United Church Publishing House, 1987.

Twitchett, Denis, and John K. Fairbank. *Cambridge History of China*. Vol. 2, Part II. Cambridge: Cambridge University Press, 1980.

Warner, Marina. *The Dragon Empress: Life and Times of Tz'u-hsi, 1835-1908, Empress Dowager of China*. London: Cardinal, 1974.

Woodham-Smith, Cecil. *Florence Nightingale, 1820-1910*. London: Fontana/Collins, 1964.

Index

Page numbers in italic indicate a figure or table. The letter "n" following a page number indicates a note; if necessary, a note number is added: for example, "11n.2" indicates note 2 on page 11.